Sponsored by the
European Association of Neurosurgical Societies

Advances and Technical Standards in Neurosurgery

Edited by

H. Krayenbühl, Zürich (Managing Editor)
J. Brihaye, Bruxelles
F. Loew, Homburg/Saar
V. Logue, London
S. Mingrino, Padova
B. Pertuiset, Paris
L. Symon, London
H. Troupp, Helsinki
M. G. Yaşargil, Zürich

Volume 6

Springer-Verlag
Wien New York 1979

With 79 Figures

Library of Congress Catalog Card Number 74-10499

Printed in Austria

ISBN 3-211-81518-X Springer-Verlag Wien — New York
ISBN 0-387-81518-X Springer-Verlag New York — Wien

Preface

As an addition to the European postgraduate training system for young neurosurgeons we began to publish in 1974 this series devoted to Advances and Technical Standards in Neurosurgery which was later sponsored by the European Association of Neurosurgical Societies.

The fact that the English language is well on the way to becoming the international medium at European scientific conferences is a great asset in terms of mutual understanding. Therefore we have decided to publish all contributions in English, regardless of the native language of the authors.

All contributions are submitted to the entire editorial board before publication of any volume.

Our series is not intended to compete with the publications of original scientific papers in other neurosurgical journals. Our intention is, rather, to present fields of neurosurgery and related areas in which important recent advances have been made. The contributions are written by specialists in the given fields and constitute the first part of each volume.

In the second part of each volume, we publish detailed descriptions of standard operative procedures, furnished by experienced clinicians; in these articles the authors describe the techniques they employ and explain the advantages, difficulties and risks involved in the various procedures. This part is intended primarily to assist young neurosurgeons in their postgraduate training. However, we are convinced that it will also be useful to experienced, fully trained neurosurgeons.

The descriptions of standard operative procedures are a novel feature of our series, and in this it differs from the similarly entitled series "Progress in Neurological Surgery"; also, our series will be mainly, but not exclusively, a forum for European neurosurgeons. We intend as well to make available the findings of European neurosurgeons which are published in less familiar languages to neurosurgeons beyond the boundaries of the authors' countries and of Europe, and we aim to promote contacts among European neurosurgeons.

We hope that neurosurgeons not only in Europe, but throughout the world, will profit by this series of "Advances and Technical Standards in Neurosurgery".

The Editors

Contents

A. Advances

B. Technical Standards

List of Contributors

Backlund, Prof. Dr. E. O., Chief of the Stereotactic Service, Department of Neurosurgery, Karolinska Hospital, S-10401 Stockholm, Sweden.

Balagura, S., M.D., Department of Neurological Surgery, Albert Einstein College of Medicine, Yeshiva University, 1300 Morris Park Avenue, Bronx, NY 10461, U.S.A.

Braakman, Prof. Dr. R., Afdeling Neurochirurgie, Academisch Ziekenhuis Rotterdam-Dijkzigt, Dr. Molewaterplein 40, Rotterdam-3002, The Netherlands.

Brihaye, Prof. Dr. J., Clinique Neurochirurgicale, Université Libre de Bruxelles, 1, rue Héger-Bordet, B-1000 Bruxelles, Belgium.

Derome, P., M.D., Service de Neurochirurgie, Hôpital Foch, 40, rue Worth, F-92151 Suresnes Cedex, France.

Georges, B., M.D., Service de Neurochirurgie, Hôpital Lariboisière, 2, rue Ambroise Paré, F-75010 Paris, France.

Gros, Prof. Dr. C., Centre Hospitalier Universitaire de Montpellier, Clinique Neuro-Chirurgicale, Centre Gui de Chauliac, F-34059 Montpellier Cedex, France.

Guiot, G., M.D., Service de Neurochirurgie, Hôpital Foch, 40, rue Worth, F-92151 Suresnes Cedex, France.

Isamat, Dr. F., Servicio de Neurocirugía, Torras y Pujalt, 1, Barcelona 22, Spain.

Kahan-Coppens, L., M.D., Service de Médecine Interne et Laboratoire d'Investigation Clinique H. J. Tagnon (Section des Maladies Infectieuses), Institut Jules Bordet, Centre des Tumeurs de l'Université Libre de Bruxelles, 1, rue Héger-Bordet, B-1000 Bruxelles, Belgium.

Klastersky, Prof. Dr. J., Service de Médecine Interne, Institut Jules Bordet, Centre des Tumeurs de l'Université Libre de Bruxelles, 1, rue Héger-Bordet, B-1000 Bruxelles, Belgium.

Porta, M., M.D., Service de Neurochirurgie, Hôpital de la Salpêtrière, 83, Boulevard de l'Hôpital, F-75634 Paris Cedex 13, France.

Visot, A., M.D., Service de Neurochirurgie, Hôpital Foch, 40, rue Worth, F-92151 Suresnes Cedex, France.

A. Advances

Stereotactic Radiosurgery in Intracranial Tumours and Vascular Malformations

E.-O. Backlund

Department of Neurosurgery, Karolinska Hospital, Stockholm (Sweden)

With 19 Figures

Contents

Introduction

In spite of the recent advances in brain surgery, the operative treatment of many intracranial conditions still offers great technical difficulties. The use of the operating microscope, especially in dextrous hands, considerably increases the possibility of achieving gratifying clinical results, but nevertheless the removal of some brain tumours, even benign, is still attended by considerable risks. Furthermore, arteriovenous malformations may if deep-seated be practically inaccessible to conventional techniques. These technical problems, inherent in traditional operations lend a sense of urgency to the development of new therapeutic methods.

In 1951, Leksell introduced the concept of "radiosurgery" and described a technique for stereotactically directing narrow beams of ionizing radiation to a limited target area within the brain without opening the skull (Leksell 1951). A new branch of the stereotactic surgery, "closed stereotactic operations", was thus established (Leksell 1971).

One of the principles of radiosurgery is that the radiation energy is delivered as a single dose to sharply circumscribed and precisely defined areas of tissue. This is possible if the radiophysical properties of the radiation sources are such that the dose gradient is very steep at the margins of the area chosen for irradiation. This, combined with precise anatomical definition of that area minimizes the side effects of the radiation. Thus, a dose can be given which is sufficient to cause necrosis of the area selected. Radiation can of course also be delivered to such an area by inserting radionuclides via a burrhole. However, when the concept "radiosurgery" was introduced, the "closed" technique was intended. In the present Chapter, the terms "radiosurgery" and "radiosurgical" will be used in this more limited sense.

The first clinical applications of radiosurgery were made with relatively low energy x-rays (Leksell *et al.* 1955) and later a well collimated proton beam (Larsson *et al.* 1958) was used for crossfire to deep structures of the brain, such as thalamic nuclei. It was suggested that this technique might also be used for the destruction of any area of tissue within the cranial compartment.

The aim of the present Chapter is to describe the radiosurgical techniques in use and the clinical experience hitherto gained during treatment of intracranial tumours and vascular malformations at the Radiosurgical Units of the Sophiahemmet Hospital and of the Stereotactic Service, Department of Neurosurgery, Karolinska Hospital, Stockholm, Sweden. Recently published case material is presented in a summarized form, but each group is illustrated with one or two representative cases from the author's personal experience, described in more detail.

At Harvard University, Boston, Massachusetts, stereotactic techniques are used for single dose treatment, predominantly for pituitary tumours and vascular malformations (Kjellberg and Kliman 1973). This group utilizes the so called "Bragg peak" of the proton beam to improve the radiophysical conditions.

Proton irradiation has also been used in the Soviet Union. An extensive study of the possibilities of achieving pituitary destruction in cases of advanced cancer has recently been published (Minakova 1977).

Lawrence and coworkers at the Donner Laboratories in Berkeley, California, have used a proton beam for irradiation of pituitary tumours since 1957; stereotactic measures are not used during these procedures, however.

Recently, 349 patients with pituitary tumours treated by this technique were reported (Lawrence *et al.* 1976).

Technique

The radiosurgical part of the Leksell system used in the present series is the "Gamma-Unit", shown in Fig. 1. The radiophysical measurements and calculations have been made by Sarby and Larsson (1965) and Dahlin *et al.* (1970).

The irradiation is performed by cross-fire to the target region with 179 narrow beams of Cobalt-60 gamma radiation distributed within a

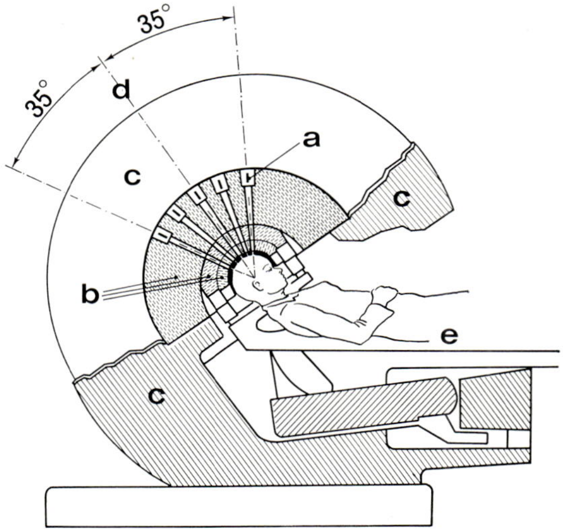

Fig. 1. Section through the Gamma Unit showing five of the beam channels. *a* ^{60}Co source, *b* collimator helmets, *c* shielding material, *d* central beam, *e* movable operating table

spherical sector. The beams are radially directed towards the centre of a collimator helmet, in which the predetermined tumour target point is positioned. At this point, the "effective radiation field" covers a very small area (Fig. 2).

As already mentioned, the technique was primarily developed for functional radiosurgery, such as thalamotomy. Because of this, the first Gamma Unit, called Unit I, was designed to give disc-shaped brain lesions with very steep dose gradients corresponding to the border zones of the lesions. For the treatment of pathological areas of tissue, however, such a dose distribution may be too small to be optimal. In order to adapt the irradiated volume to the shape of a tumour, for example, a number of target points in a predetermined spatial pattern can be utilized. To achieve even bigger fields of radiation and of spherical shape, another Gamma Unit with wider distribution of the radioactive sources and cylindrical apertures for each individual beam was designed (Unit II).

If the number and the spatial distribution of the cobalt sources are varied the "shape" of the summated dose distribution around the target point can be correspondingly altered. In Unit II it is possible to extinguish optionally any of the 179 sources by simply plugging the collimator channels, which allows the dose distribution, within certain limits, to be more or less "tailor-made" to the individual case. For this modification, a computer (PDP 11) is used. The calculation technique has been described by Arndt *et al.* (1975).

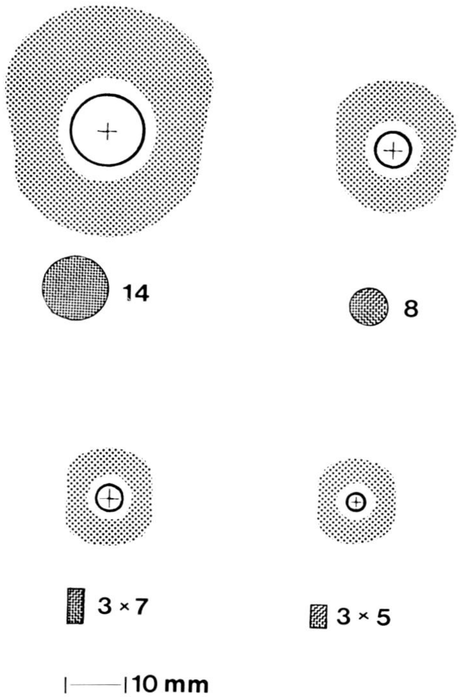

Fig. 2. Isodose diagrams in A-P plane at the centre of a human head: In Unit II the cross section of each individual beam is circular and can be varied to 14 and 8 mms in diameter, respectively. The dose distributions for these two collimator alternatives are shown in the upper row. In Unit I the cross section of each beam is 3 × 7 or 3 × 5 mm, respectively. These two alternatives are shown in the lower row. The black circular line of each dose diagram corresponds to the 90% isodose level and the dotted area to the 10 to 50% isodose level. The 100% level is at the centre (indicated by a cross)

The radiation doses mentioned in the following are, if not otherwise mentioned, expressed in terms of "target dose", *i.e.* the dose at the stereotactic target point, in the tumour cases as a rule identical with the centre of the tumour. The relative isodose levels are expressed in per cent of this target dose (dose maximum). A spatial agreement between the tumour surface and the 50% isodose level has been aimed at, in general.

The radiosurgical procedure including the determination of the stereotactic coordinates is intrinsically safe provided that the area chosen for destruction is either visible itself or can be spatially related to visible reference structures on the stereotactic films. As an example of the latter case, our experiences include attempts at indirect localization of pituitary microadenomas by studying discrete changes of the sella turcica. Examples of making target areas visible are those of stereotactic cisternography using positive contrast (acoustic tumours) and stereotactic angiography (arterio-venous malformations).

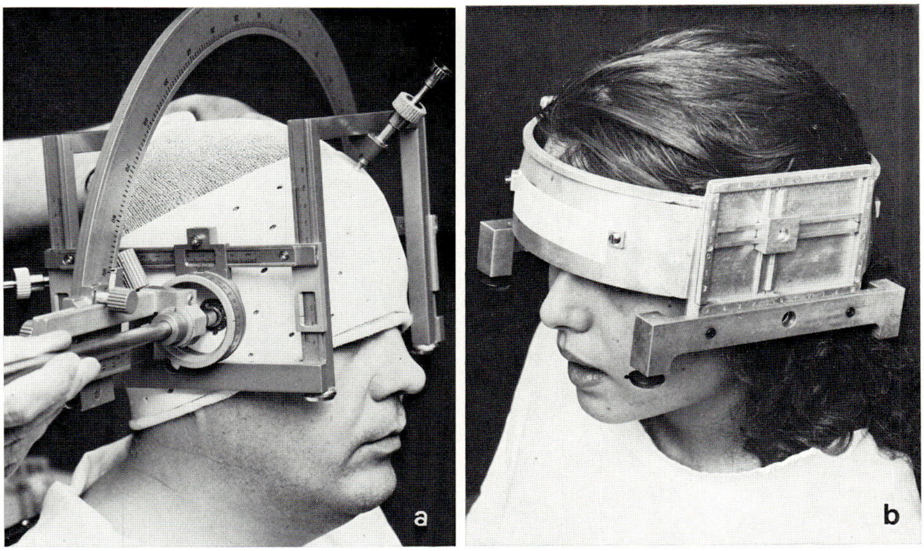

Fig. 3. The patient is fixed to the Gamma Unit by one of two methods: a) A thermoplast ("Orthoplast") is modelled around the patient's head. According to the stereotactic coordinates, metal bearings are attached, fitting to movable fixation axes of the collimator helmet. b) A circular metallic frame is secured to the skull by four screws and bearings on each side of the frame are adjusted according to the coordinates

Of equal importance is the technique for fastening the patient in the Gamma Unit's collimator helmet. At present, two alternative techniques are in use; either a well-fitting plastic cap is modelled around the patient's head, or a metallic fixture is applied to it by screws secured to the skull (Figs. 3 a and b).

The principles and the techniques of stereotaxy are related in a natural way to computed tomography (CT). This has been utilized in our practice.

The major practical and mechanical problems of aligning the scanner geometry to the stereotactic system have been solved (Greitz *et al.* 1975, Bergström and Greitz 1976). In a number of cases including pinealomas, acoustic tumours and retinoblastomas, stereotactic CT technique has been used. The target point of the area to be irradiated is selected on the CT-display, and its stereotactic coordinates are determined by the computer of the scanner (Fig. 4). This technique is now under further development.

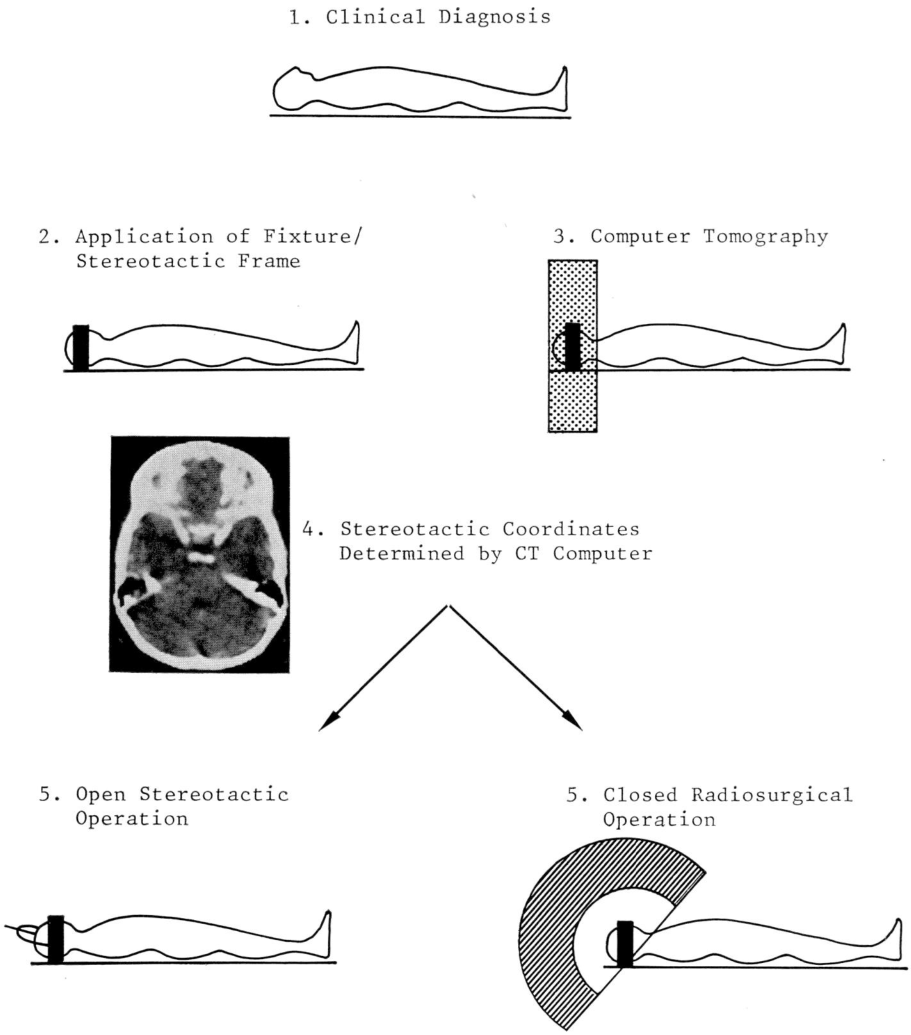

Fig. 4. Coordinate determination by computed tomography preceeding the stereotactic procedure: The patient's head fixture is secured in the CT-scanner whereby the stereotactic coordinates can be obtained by the computer of the scanner. The method is used optionally prior to either open stereotactic operations or closed radiosurgery

In concluding this section, the simplicity of the radiosurgical technique as compared with the painstaking and often tedious conventional operations should be emphasized. The patients reported in this presentation have as a rule been treated under slight pre-medication only, and in a number of cases, the radiosurgery was even performed entirely as an out-patient procedure.

Acoustic Tumours

In skilled hands, microsurgical techniques offer the possibility of radically removing acoustic neurinomas of small or moderate size with minimal risk of postoperative deficits or fatal outcome. It is doubtful, however, if the average neurosurgeon will ever have the chance to achieve results comparable to those obtained at selected centers, where problems of acoustic surgery are the dominant interest. The necessity for alternative non-invasive methods of treatment is thus obvious.

In 1969 the first patient with an acoustic neurinoma was treated by radiosurgery (Leksell 1971). She was a young woman with von Recklinghausen's disease and bilateral tumours for which surgical intervention was not considered advisable. The tumour on her right side was treated with a target dose of 70 Gy. Careful follow-up of this patient showed conclusively that the growth of the treated tumour was arrested and a decrease of its size was even found at a recent follow-up 8 years after the irradiation. Her left tumour was treated in Unit II in 1975. With the exception of a pronounced hearing deficiency, she is now in good condition and has full working capacity nine years after the first irradiation.

A second pilot case was treated in 1969. This patient had a large tumour, but refused conventional surgery. Radiosurgery was performed with the radiation field covering only the tumour's central region. When papilledema appeared two years later, the patient accepted surgery and an intracapsular tumour removal was performed. In the operative specimen necrotic changes were found indicating a centrally located radiation injury.

During the years 1971–1974, seven more patients were treated. All had medium-sized or small tumours. They were treated with Unit I and several targets had to be used in six cases; the aim was to achieve at least 50% of the target dose within the borders of the tumour. The stereotactic localization was based upon morphological information obtained from the preoperative air encephalography, and the internal meatus was used as the reference structure. In one case of a young woman who was treated after open surgery (intracapsular removal), the postoperative tumour anatomy necessary for the dose planning was difficult to outline. In one more case, an optimal agreement between the radiation field and the full extent of the tumour was possibly not achieved. The tumours of both these patients increased in size and were re-irradiated in Unit II. Both are in good condition at present.

The other five cases which constitute a homogeneous group have recently (November 1977) been examined clinically and with positive contrast cisternography. After an average observation time of more than four years, these five patients are in perfect condition, and in all cases but one shrinkage of the tumour has been demonstrated. In the remaining case the tumour size was unchanged. The facial nerve function is normal in all cases. One patient complains of a slight facial sensory deficit which is difficult to explain. In two cases, increased hearing was found at the follow-up. A detailed record of these nine cases is under preparation at present (Norén *et al.* 1979).

side was 0.1 and on the left 1.0. Her visual field on the left side was normal, and on the right side there was a nasal defect for minor objects, Computed tomography showed a 4 × 4 cm suprasellar expanding lesion, most probably entirely solid (Fig. 9 a). The attenuation was enhanced after intravenous contrast injection.

When planning the radiosurgery it was obvious that even with the use of the biggest collimator system of Unit II, an optimal correlation between the tumour volume and the radiation field could not be obtained. Since, however, no other therapeutic alternative was conceivable, a radiolesion was placed in the basal two-thirds of the tumour. The target dose was 50 Gy

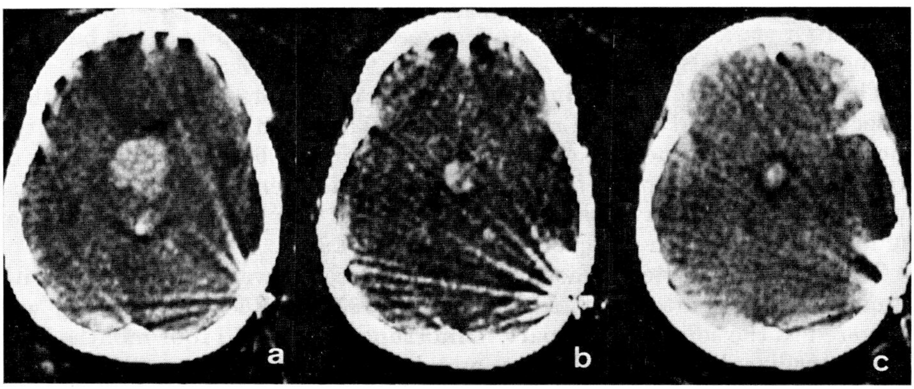

Fig. 9 a, b, and c. Case CRA 39: Computed tomography of a solid craniopharyngioma a) before the treatment, b) half a year later and c) one year and a half after radiosurgery

but the most peripheral part of the tumour did not receive more than about 5 Gy. Immediately postoperatively the patient had a headache, which was assumed to be due to radiation induced edema of the tumour. Support for this theory was gained as the symptoms disappeared promptly after administration of dexamethazone. On the third postoperative day the patient went back to her home hospital for further careful observation.

The patient came back for control in July 1976. She considered herself then completely healthy. Computed tomography showed a considerable decrease of the tumour size (Fig. 9 b). Its diameter was estimated to 1.6 cm. The patient returned for another CT control in May 1977 when a further decrease was registered, the tumour diameter was only about one cm, corresponding to a 60-fold volume decrease (Fig. 9 c). The tumour was surrounded by wide cisterns. The third ventricle was not well seen due to artefacts from the shunt, but the anterior horns of the lateral ventricles appeared normal. The visual acuity was slightly improved and the right visual field was normal.

Conclusions

The treatment of craniopharyngiomas by attempted radical removal still poses problems and stereotactic puncture should therefore be consistently included in the diagnostic management of these tumours. The

Acoustic Tumours

In skilled hands, microsurgical techniques offer the possibility of radically removing acoustic neurinomas of small or moderate size with minimal risk of postoperative deficits or fatal outcome. It is doubtful, however, if the average neurosurgeon will ever have the chance to achieve results comparable to those obtained at selected centers, where problems of acoustic surgery are the dominant interest. The necessity for alternative non-invasive methods of treatment is thus obvious.

In 1969 the first patient with an acoustic neurinoma was treated by radiosurgery (Leksell 1971). She was a young woman with von Recklinghausen's disease and bilateral tumours for which surgical intervention was not considered advisable. The tumour on her right side was treated with a target dose of 70 Gy. Careful follow-up of this patient showed conclusively that the growth of the treated tumour was arrested and a decrease of its size was even found at a recent follow-up 8 years after the irradiation. Her left tumour was treated in Unit II in 1975. With the exception of a pronounced hearing deficiency, she is now in good condition and has full working capacity nine years after the first irradiation.

A second pilot case was treated in 1969. This patient had a large tumour, but refused conventional surgery. Radiosurgery was performed with the radiation field covering only the tumour's central region. When papilledema appeared two years later, the patient accepted surgery and an intracapsular tumour removal was performed. In the operative specimen necrotic changes were found indicating a centrally located radiation injury.

During the years 1971–1974, seven more patients were treated. All had medium-sized or small tumours. They were treated with Unit I and several targets had to be used in six cases; the aim was to achieve at least 50% of the target dose within the borders of the tumour. The stereotactic localization was based upon morphological information obtained from the preoperative air encephalography, and the internal meatus was used as the reference structure. In one case of a young woman who was treated after open surgery (intracapsular removal), the postoperative tumour anatomy necessary for the dose planning was difficult to outline. In one more case, an optimal agreement between the radiation field and the full extent of the tumour was possibly not achieved. The tumours of both these patients increased in size and were re-irradiated in Unit II. Both are in good condition at present.

The other five cases which constitute a homogeneous group have recently (November 1977) been examined clinically and with positive contrast cisternography. After an average observation time of more than four years, these five patients are in perfect condition, and in all cases but one shrinkage of the tumour has been demonstrated. In the remaining case the tumour size was unchanged. The facial nerve function is normal in all cases. One patient complains of a slight facial sensory deficit which is difficult to explain. In two cases, increased hearing was found at the follow-up. A detailed record of these nine cases is under preparation at present (Norén *et al.* 1979).

Since 1975, when Unit II was put into use, a further series of 28 patients has been treated. A more homogeneous dose distribution was possible with this unit, but on the other hand, the dose gradient was not as sharp and the surrounding structures may have received a larger fraction of the dose. Preliminary investigations including repeated CT-scans (Norén and Backlund 1977) indicate arrested tumour growth in all cases but three. In many cases, areas of decreased attenuation on CT-scan have been found in the central part of the tumour, these correspond spatially to the area irradiated, and probably indicate destroyed tissue. Some untoward effects have been encountered; transient facial nerve paresis suddenly appeared approximately half a year after the treatment in ten cases. In seven cases, sensory disturbances in the face occurred. All these side-effects were seen predominantly in the age group over 60 years.

As neurilemmoma tissue has been assumed to be radio-resistant, heavy doses have been used up to now. The appropriate dose level has now to be established and the undesirable side-effects carefully analyzed. The preoperative assessment in the next series will include studies concerning the individual tumour growth rate and histological classification by stereotactic biopsy (Fig. 5).

Case Report (ACU **7***)*

A 55-year old man was examined at another hospital in 1971 because of two year's hearing deficiency. Widening of the right internal meatus was found although air encephalography was found to be normal. A new air study was performed in the autumn of 1972 which revealed a tumour in the right cerebello-pontine angle; its size was 1.3 cm in diameter. The patient was sent to our department for assessment and radiosurgery.

On admission he presented a normal neurologic state with the exception of the right-sided hearing loss. Audiologic examination revealed a hearing threshold elevation, indicating a retrocochlear injury. Stapedius reflex test and tone decay test indicated a retrocochlear localization. There was no caloric reaction. In June 1973 the tumour was irradiated in Unit I and three targets were used. The radiation dose to each target was 50 Gy and the average tumour dose was estimated to 30 Gy.

The first post-operative control after three months showed the patient's condition unchanged. An EMG of the patient's facial muscles showed a slight reduction of voluntary activity in the right orbicularis oculi muscle but no signs of denervation. In spite of these findings the functional state of his face was normal and symmetric.

In the autumn of 1974 the patient was thoroughly examined by cisternography with positive contrast and for the first time by computed tomography. The former showed that the tumour diameter now was 1.1 cm (Fig. 6 a). On the CT-scan the tumour could not be visualized, not even after intravenous contrast enhancement. The EMG was now normal. An audiologic examination revealed that the hearing function of the affected ear had improved slightly. Re-examination one year later showed the

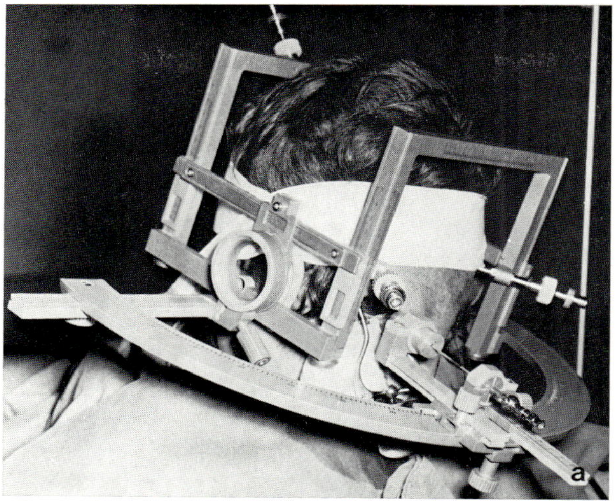

Fig. 5 a. Stereotactic biopsy from an acoustic tumour performed via a burr hole over the cerebellar hemisphere, with the patient awake and in sitting position

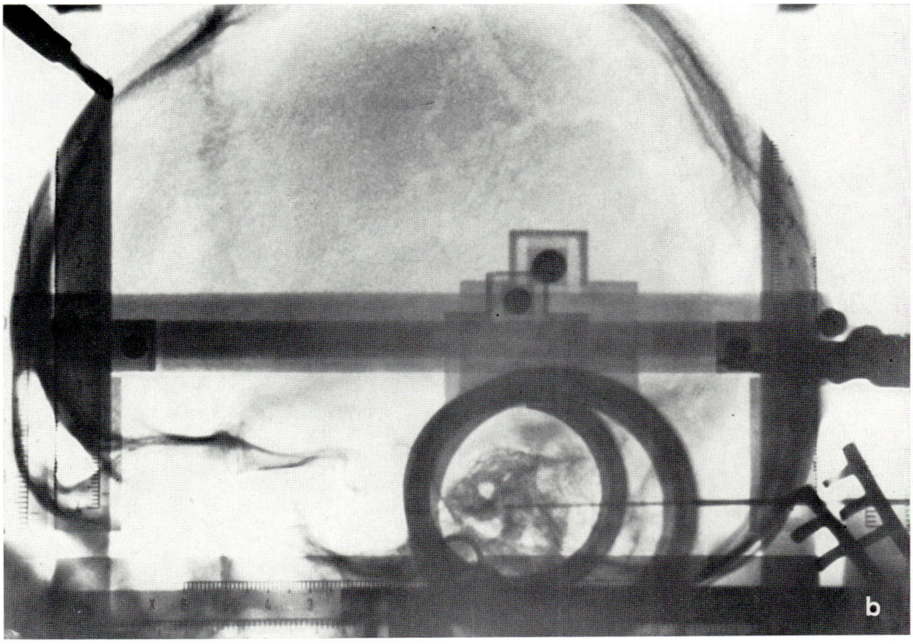

Fig. 5 b. Stereotactic film from the procedure shown in a)

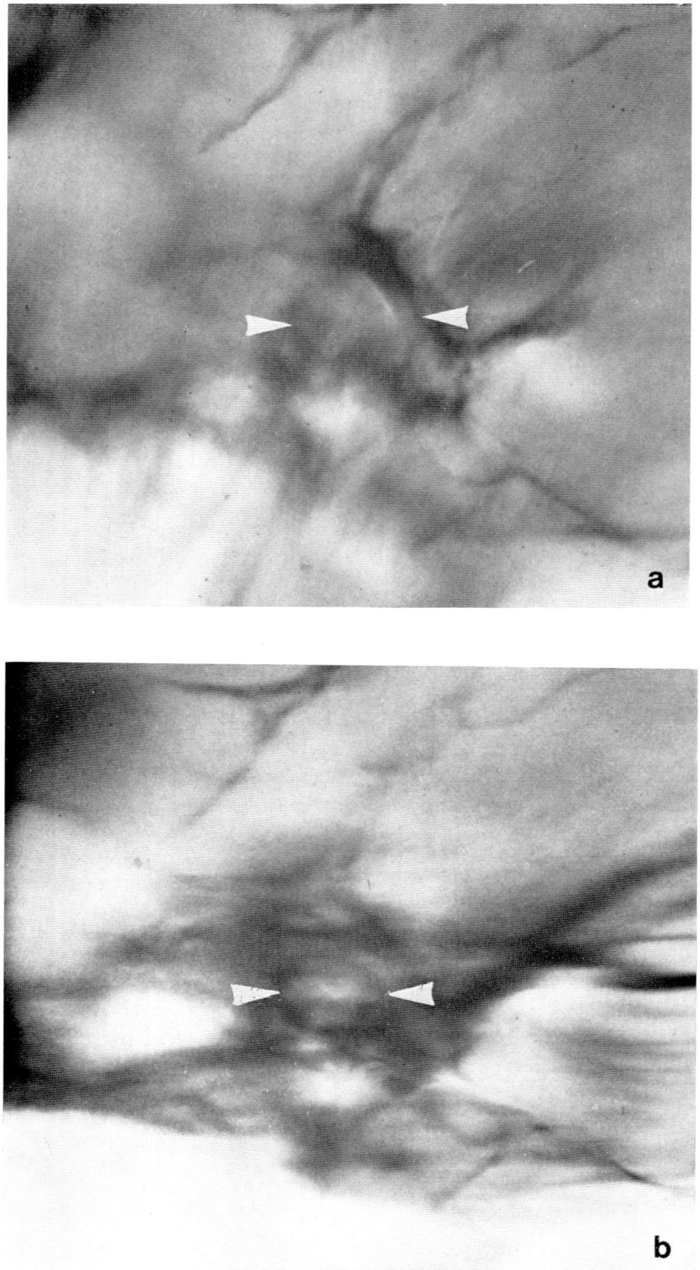

Fig. 6 a and b. Case ACU 7: Metrizamide cisternography (lateral view) a) one year and b) four years after radiosurgical treatment of an acoustic neurinoma showing shrinkage of tumour

patient's condition to be completely unchanged. The appearance of the tumour on x-ray, including cisternography and CT-scan, was the same as previously.

The most recent follow-up was in November 1977. The patient was still in an excellent condition with a normal neurologic state except the hearing loss which, on audiologic examination, was found to be less pronounced than previously. Positive contrast cisternography showed a further decrease of tumour diameter to 0.8 cm (Fig. 6 b).

Conclusions

The radiosurgical technique makes possible a radical treatment of acoustic tumours. Our preliminary results show that gradual tumour shrinkage without undesirable side-effects can be initiated by radiosurgery if the demands for a steep dose-gradient versus the tumour's surroundings are strictly respected. Clinical results from a small series of cases treated in accordance with the above-mentioned criterion are comparable with the best results reported after present open surgery.

Tumours in the Pineal Region

Tumours in the region of the pineal gland and the quadrigeminal plate are often clinically classified as "pinealomas" but their histological characteristics can vary considerably. Irrespective of their microscopic appearance, however, they may be suitable objects for radiosurgery if they are of appropriate size and can be well outlined by diagnostic x-ray studies. In each case, the ultimate choice of treatment method should be made after a stereotactic biopsy (Fig. 7). One more reason for this type of fine-needle biopsy is the possible presence of cystic lesions.

Since 1969, we have treated 13 cases by radiosurgery after attempts at cytological classification. From a pathological point of view this case

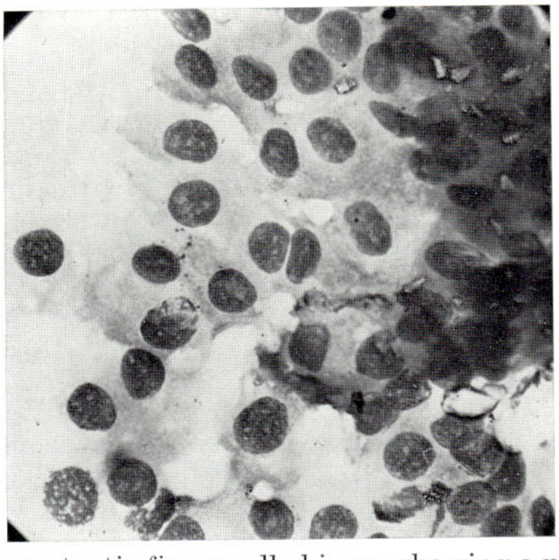

Fig. 7. Smear from a stereotactic fine needle biopsy showing a pineocytoma (Courtesy, Dr. S. Franzén)

material is very heterogeneous and in three cases even the biopsy specimen was not conclusive. Four cases were classified as pineocytomas, two as ependymomas and three as astrocytomas (Kernohan's classification). The clinical data are compiled in Table 1. The average tumour diameter varied between one and three cms and target doses of 20–75 Gy were given. Two patients died, both of whom were initially classified as pineocytomas but

Table 1. *Tumours in the Pineal Region, Treated by Radiosurgery 1969—1977*

Age/ Sex	Stereotactic biopsy	Average tumour diameter, cms	Target dose, Gy/ Irradiation date	Results
42/F	not performed	2	20/May 1969 50/Jan 1970	Lost for follow-up
13/F	pineocytoma	2	50/Aug 1969	1977 Excellent, see Case report
7/M	no exchange	1	40/Sep 1970	1976 CT: no change, 1977 excellent condition
33/F	"connective tissue"	2	50/May 1971	1976 CT: no change, 1977 excellent condition
21/M	pineocytoma	2.5	50/Apr 1972	Died 3 years later in disseminating tumour. Biopsy result erroneous?
24/F	"epithelial cells"	1.5	50/Sep 1972	Encephalography 1973: no change, 1977 excellent condition. CT not yet performed
7/M	pineocytoma	3	50/Jun 1973	Died 2 years later in medulloblastoma. Initial smears revised, found to be erroneous
29/M	ependymoma	3	75/Dec 1975	1976 CT: no tumour visible, 1977 excellent condition
64/F	ependymoma	3	50/Jan 1976	1977 CT: tumour increase. Partially disabled
9/F	astrocytoma II	2	50/Mar 1976	1977 CT: no tumour visible. Attending school
27/M	astrocytoma II	2?	70/Feb 1977	Tumour increase, additional conventional radiotherapy, 50 Gy. Partially disabled, on steroids
70/M	astrocytoma III	1.2	30/Mar 1977	1977 CT: no tumour visible
12/M	pineocytoma	2.5	20/Dec 1977	Obs. period too short

the interpretation of the initial smears was found to be erroneous at least for one who proved to harbour a medulloblastoma. In one of the astrocytoma cases additional radiotherapy was needed because of progressive tumour growth. It is questionable whether this patient should have been treated by radiosurgery, as it could not be excluded that the tumour was originating from the posterior part of thalamus. Two of the cases (13/F and 21/M in Table 1) have been published previously (Backlund *et al.* 1974), before the malignant character of the second case was disclosed.

The average observation time of this series is almost four years. The first case of the series, who was a foreigner, is lost to follow-up. Eight cases had a shunt inserted preoperatively and in two of these cases this was performed after the irradiation. The patient with the longest observation time (eight years) is described in detail below. She is, furthermore, one of those who was not subjected to a shunt operation.

Case Report (PIN 2)

A 17-year old girl was admitted in July 1969 with a one month history of attacks of headache accompanied by nausea and vomiting. Bilateral papilledema of two diopters was confirmed on admission. Encephalography revealed deformation of the posterior part of the third ventricle, suggesting a rounded pinealoma of two cms diameter (Fig. 8 a). The aqueduct was displaced and partially obstructed and marked ventricular dilatation was present. No tumour vessels were seen on vertebral angiography. Stereotactic aspiration biopsy of the tumour was performed and the cytologic appearance indicated a pineocytoma. In August 1969 the tumour was treated in Unit I. Four stereotactic target points were chosen to give a dose distribution covering the tumour. A dose of 50 Gg was delivered to each target and no part of the tumour received less than 5 Gy.

Post-operatively, the papilledema disappeared rapidly within two weeks. Simultaneously the symptoms and signs of raised intracranial pressure were relieved.

Air encephalography one year later showed the tumour region to be almost normal (Fig. 8 b) and the lateral ventricles of ordinary size and shape. The patient was then perfectly healthy and the ocular fundi were normal. A second air encephalogram three years after treatment revealed no obvious further change, although the pineal lesion was possibly still smaller.

Since treatment the patient has finished her schooling and started working as a medical attendant. She became pregnant and gave birth to a normal child in 1977. She was readmitted for control in November the same year and found to be in excellent condition. She denied having headaches, diplopia, visual field defects or unsteady gait. An neuro-ophthalmological examination was normal as was an endocrine screening. Air encephalography indicated possible further decrease of the size of the tumour remnant.

After more than eight years' follow-up with proven continuous gradual shrinkage of the tumour, the patient is now considered cured.

Conclusion

If the tumours in the pineal region are classified by stereotactic fine needle biopsy—which should be made in every case—a majority of the cases can be managed without further open surgery. Benign tumours of appropriate size and form are suitable objects for radiosurgery. The malignant varieties are properly classified and pointless surgery is avoided. The patients in this latter category can then be referred to radiotherapy without unnecessary delay. In cases with cystic lesions, the diagnostic puncture may constitute the whole therapeutic procedure.

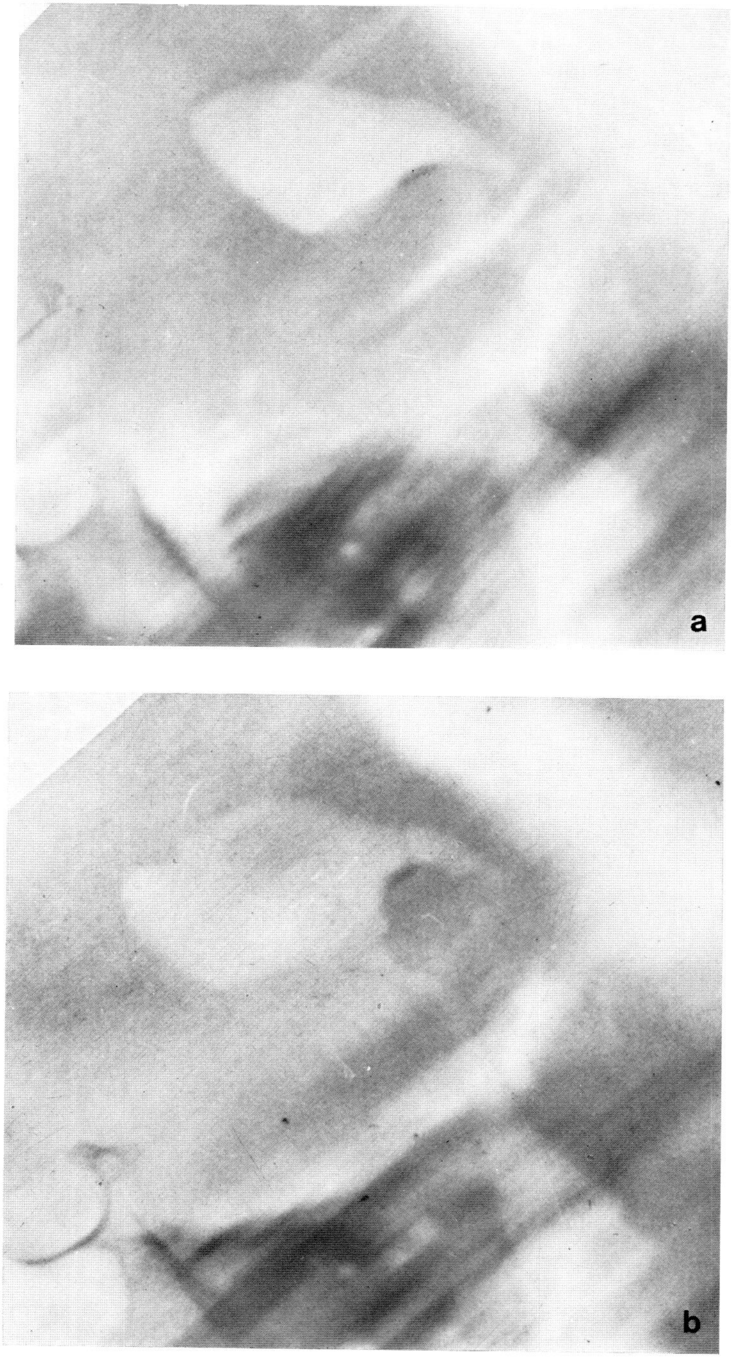

Fig. 8 a and b. Case PIN 2: Air encephalography in a case of pineocytoma, a) before and b) one year after radiosurgery

Craniopharyngiomas

In most craniopharyngioma cases the clinical symptoms are caused by expanding cysts, whereas the solid portions appear to grow slowly. A treatment which merely keeps the cystic parts under control thus solves many of the problems arising in cases of craniopharyngiomas. A program for intracystic treatment with radionuclides in colloidal solution has been developed (Backlund *et al.* 1972) and clinical results presented (Backlund 1973). As the solid tumour remnants after this therapy constitute a permanent substrate for the development of new cysts, these remnants should also be irradiated. Results from combined intracystic radionuclide and radiosurgical treatment of solid tumour parts have been obtained from a consecutive series during the last ten years and have proved to be long-lasting (Backlund 1977).

There is evidence that craniopharyngiomas are more radiosensitive than expected (Backlund 1969, Landolt 1974). This is in agreement with the "organ of origin" concept (cf. Rubin and Casarett 1968) as the histology of craniopharyngiomas resembles that of the radiosensitive oropharyngeal epithelium. After conventional radiotherapy a complete disappearance of tumour has even been reported (Kramer *et al.* 1968).

The first case treated radiosurgically in our series was a young man with tumour remnants after cyst treatment. In 1967, a single dose of 20 Gy was delivered to the solid tumour part. Unfortunately he died four months later from tonsillar herniation due to an obstruction in the ventriculoatrial shunt. The autopsy showed extensive destruction of the tumour (Backlund 1969).

Subsequently, 11 additional cases have been treated by the same technique, which constitute about 15% of all craniopharyngiomas treated in our service since radiosurgery became available. In eight of these, tumour remnants after various other forms of therapy were irradiated, but in three cases, the radiosurgical treatment was the first therapeutic measure. The doses have varied between 20 and 50 Gy and the average observation time is approximately four years. No undue side effects attributable to the treatment have been recorded.

Case Report (CRA 39)

A 39-year old Finnish lady had had two normal pregnancies and normal menstruation up to 1972 when amenorrhea appeared. One year later the patient noticed transient impaired vision. She was then examined at her home hospital by technetium scintigraphy which showed a slight uptake in the suprasellar region. For unknown reasons further investigations were postponed until 1975 when thorough neuroradiology disclosed a very large tumour in the hypothalamic region. The sella turcica was of normal size and appearance. A shunt was then installed, and stereotactic biopsy from the tumour revealed a solid craniopharyngioma. The tumour was considered inoperable and the patient was sent to our department for radiosurgery.

On admission in December 1975 the patient's visual acuity on the right side was 0.1 and on the left 1.0. Her visual field on the left side was normal, and on the right side there was a nasal defect for minor objects, Computed tomography showed a 4 × 4 cm suprasellar expanding lesion, most probably entirely solid (Fig. 9 a). The attenuation was enhanced after intravenous contrast injection.

When planning the radiosurgery it was obvious that even with the use of the biggest collimator system of Unit II, an optimal correlation between the tumour volume and the radiation field could not be obtained. Since, however, no other therapeutic alternative was conceivable, a radiolesion was placed in the basal two-thirds of the tumour. The target dose was 50 Gy

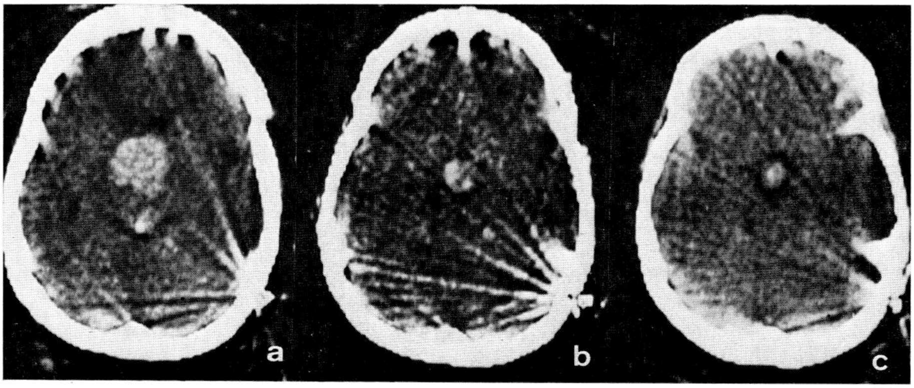

Fig. 9 a, b, and c. Case CRA 39: Computed tomography of a solid craniopharyngioma a) before the treatment, b) half a year later and c) one year and a half after radiosurgery

but the most peripheral part of the tumour did not receive more than about 5 Gy. Immediately postoperatively the patient had a headache, which was assumed to be due to radiation induced edema of the tumour. Support for this theory was gained as the symptoms disappeared promptly after administration of dexamethazone. On the third postoperative day the patient went back to her home hospital for further careful observation.

The patient came back for control in July 1976. She considered herself then completely healthy. Computed tomography showed a considerable decrease of the tumour size (Fig. 9 b). Its diameter was estimated to 1.6 cm. The patient returned for another CT control in May 1977 when a further decrease was registered, the tumour diameter was only about one cm, corresponding to a 60-fold volume decrease (Fig. 9 c). The tumour was surrounded by wide cisterns. The third ventricle was not well seen due to artefacts from the shunt, but the anterior horns of the lateral ventricles appeared normal. The visual acuity was slightly improved and the right visual field was normal.

Conclusions

The treatment of craniopharyngiomas by attempted radical removal still poses problems and stereotactic puncture should therefore be consistently included in the diagnostic management of these tumours. The

During radiosurgery, two cases received 70 and 50 Gy respectively to a target point at the centre of the anterior lobe. In the third case—with the asymmetric sella—the dose maximum was placed in the right part of the lobe.

As in the Cushing group, a gradual normalization was found in all patients after the treatment. After an observation time of 25 to 30 months, the hyperpigmentation was found to be considerably reduced in two cases and completely absent in one.

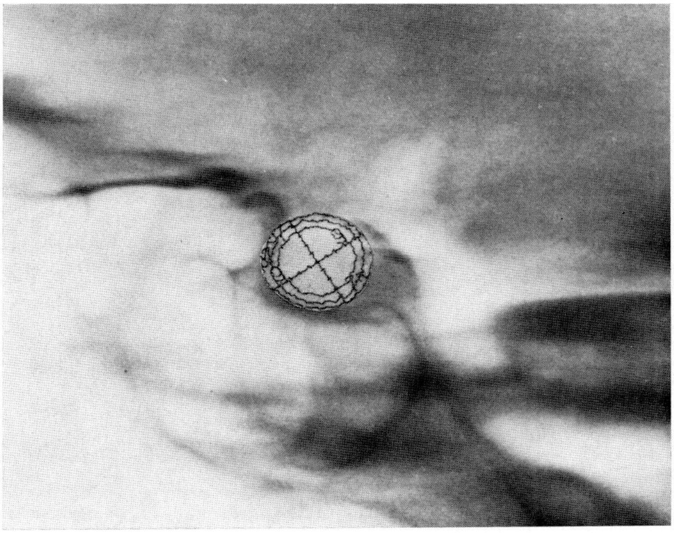

Fig. 11. Case CUS 5: In this patient with Cushing's disease and a normal sella turcica the display from the dose planning computer is superimposed upon the x-ray film. The three circular lines correspond to the 90, 70 and 50% isodose levels (Unit II). The optic pathways are assumed to be situated well outside the 10% isodose level

In one of the Nelson cases, which received 70 Gy, a very small, unilateral visual field defect appeared one year after the treatment. The patient had not noticed it, due to her previous history of glaucoma. Control air encephalography was performed and showed that the volume of the sellar contents had decreased and that the preoperative slight herniation of the suprasellar cisterns had increased. It must be noted, that the radiation dose to the optic pathways in this case was calculated to be less than the dose to corresponding structures in the other cases treated. A possible explanation might be that the impairment was due to a radiation injury to some of the tiny arteries supplying the optic pathways from beneath, or to traction on the optic nerves when the cisternal herniation increased.

Case Report (CUS 5)

The patient was a 40-year old woman with normal and regular menstruation who had had three normal pregnancies before the onset of her illness, the most recent 8 years before admission. At that time an arterial hypertension was found which gradually became therapy-resistant. Concomitantly, the patient noticed a continuous weight gain and the appearance of a "buffalo hump". She developed hirsutism, striae and an increased tendency for bruises. In 1974 the patient had a mental depression which was medically treated.

On admission in October 1975 the patient's face was rosy and of a "moon face appearance" (Fig. 12 a). The subcutaneous fat was increased in the dorsocervical and supraclavicular regions. Hirsutism and striae as

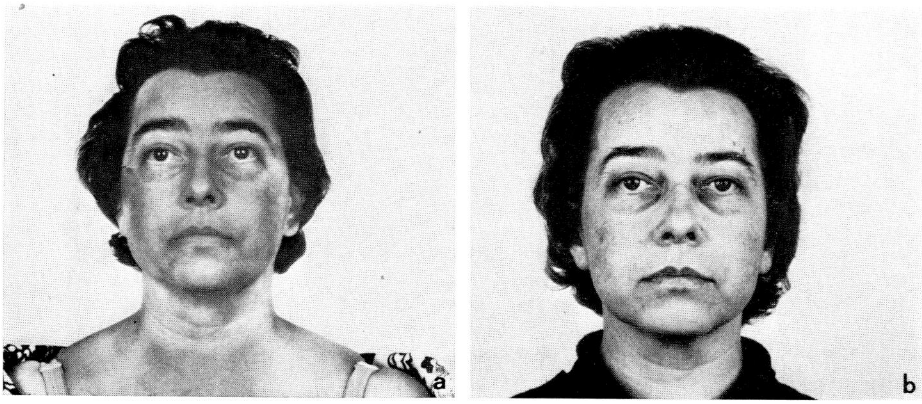

Fig. 12 a and b. Case CUS 5 (cf. Fig. 11): a) before and b) two years after radiosurgical treatment

well as a slight hyperpigmentation were found. Extremities were slim and her blood pressure was 180/110.

The diagnosis of a pituitary-dependent Cushing's syndrome was made after laboratory examination.

Aortography showed no tumour of the adrenals. Skull x-ray revealed a normal sella turcica, but with possible slight asymmetry. Preoperative pneumoencephalography showed no suprasellar mass. On the contrary, a slight herniation of the suprasellar cisterns was found.

Radiosurgery was performed in late 1975 when 70 Gy were delivered to a target point located in the medial-inferior part of the anterior lobe. At least 50% of the adenohypophysis (*i.e.* the central part) received more than 90% of the target dose (Fig. 11).

After the operation, the patient's symptoms disappeared gradually and the laboratory findings returned to normal. At the two year follow-up she had a normalized circadian rhythm of plasma cortisol, the urinary cortiols values were 75–110 nmol/24 H and normal suppression of glucocorticoid production occurred after dexamethasone. The patient's typical Cushing appearance had by then completely disappeared (Fig. 12 b) and her blood pressure was 130–160/80–90 mm Hg.

2. *Acromegaly*

In those acromegalic states suspected of being caused by microadenomas, results as satisfactory as in the above-mentioned Cushing and Nelson series should be expected. Unfortunately, with few exceptions, the acromegalic cases admitted to our department have had tumours too large for radiosurgical treatment. In eight pilot cases treated in Unit I with a follow-up of 6–7 years, the results have been varied, but in general less successful than those reported after proton beam treatment (Kjellberg and Kliman 1973, Lawrence *et al.* 1976). In most of the cases, however, an early but transient decrease of the acromegalic symptoms was noticed sometimes combined with lowered growth hormone (GH) values. Some cases, initially classified as failures, displayed a clinical cure and even hypopituitarism after several years. The collective experience from this series speaks in favour of using stereotactic radiosurgery for small GH producing adenomas. Refined diagnostic methods, in combination with the improved irradiation technique now available, may lead to results after radiosurgery comparable to the excellent results obtained after selective adenomectomy (Hardy and Vezina 1976).

Two of the cases from the pilot series mentioned above followed an interesting course and are described here. In Case I, a lasting cure was obtained after irradiation with only 20 Gy to a minute area, suspected of harbouring a microadenoma. In the second case, the bulk of the tumour was diminished but the effect upon the acromegaly was transient; only the intrasellar part of the large intra- and suprasellar tumour seemed to be responsible for the GH hypersecretion.

Case Report I (ACR 1)

The patient was a 58-year old woman with a 10 year history of acromegaly which had been previously treated with conventional x-rays without effect. Her serum GH level was pathologically high. X-rays of the skull showed a sella turcica that was only moderately enlarged, but its form was such that a microadenoma situated in its most anterior part was suspected. Pneumoencephalography showed no suprasellar extension. Transsphenoidal surgery was discussed but was considered too risky because of the patient's severe therapy resistant arterial hypertension and secondary cardiac failure. It was decided to treat the patient by radiosurgery. Because of her previous radiotherapy, 20 Gy was delivered to a very small field in the anterior part of the sella turcica adjacent to a local bulging of the sellar floor (Fig. 13). This treatment had a dramatic effect upon her blood pressure which normalized within 2 weeks, and the patient even developed an orthostatic hypotension (Fig. 14). This was thought to be a result of a secondary adrenal insufficiency due to an acute radiation-induced hypopituitarism, but the plasma cortisol proved to be normal and the hypotension could not be explained. Simultaneously, the symptoms of acromegaly began to disappear and the GH values became normal. Later on, the hypertension gradually reappeared, but the symptoms of acromegaly have remained absent during an observation time of more than eight years. Her serum GH level at a recent control was 4 ng/mg.

Case Report II (ACR 6)

A 40-year old man was admitted in 1969 who had 10 years' history of classical acromegaly. Two years previously a considerably enlarged sella turcica had been found. One year later he developed homonymous quandrantic hemianopia and air encephalography was performed. This showed a large intra- and suprasellar expanding lesion, which displaced the anterior

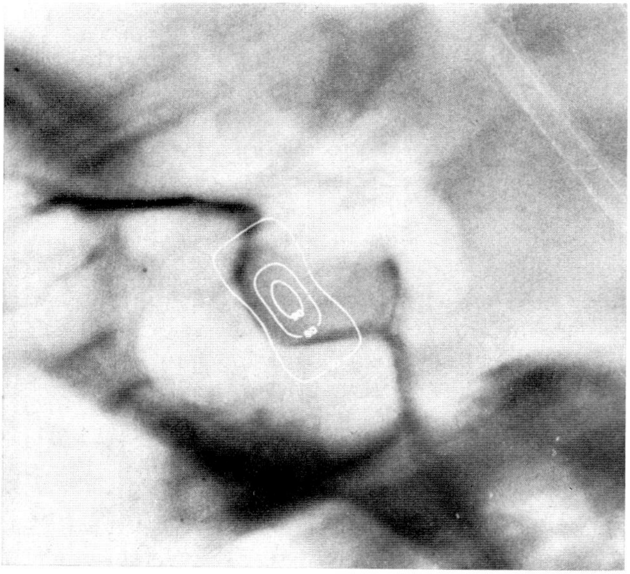

Fig. 13. Case ACR 1: In this acromegalic patient a microadenoma was suspected in the anterior part of the sella turcica. The isodose curves (Unit I) are superimposed upon the x-ray film. The irradiated area is indicated by the 90, 50 and 10% levels

part of the third ventricle backwards and upwards (Fig. 15 a). The visual acuity of the right eye was 1.0 and of the left 0.1. The average GH level was pathologically high.

In April 1969 the intrasellar tumour area was treated in Unit I. Four targets were used and 15 Gy were given to each target. The patient experienced an immediate subjective improvement. There was no obvious objective decrease of his acromegalic activity except that he was able to remove his finger ring, which had been impossible for years. The GH values were unchanged.

In October of the same year the patient came back for treatment of the suprasellar tumour part. On that admission the patient was very eager to emphasize a definite subjective improvement during the months prior to admission. He could speak more easily and had less sweating and less pronounced paraesthesiae. The suprasellar tumour portion was then irradiated with a dose of 50 Gy to each of five targets.

Frequent examination of this patient showed an unchanged endocrine status during the next three years. In 1971, the patient grew worse again but one year later air encephalography showed that the tumour was smaller than previously. The visual fields and visual acuity were unchanged. The GH level was somewhat lower but still pathologically high. The suprasellar tumour portion was considered adequately treated, whereas the intrasellar part, probably responsible for the GH production, was obviously insufficiently treated. Additional irradiation was planned in Unit II, which was at that time under construction.

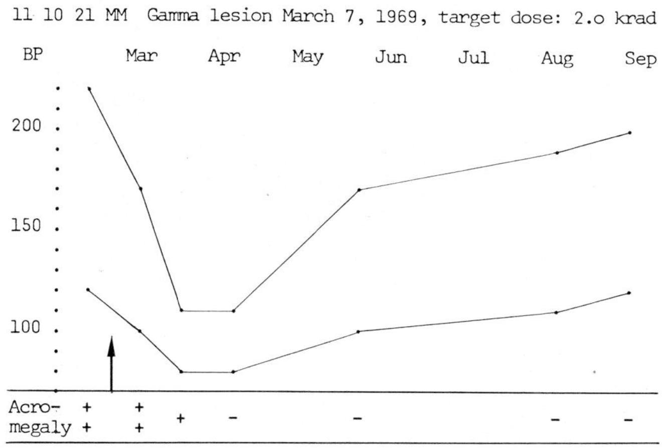

Fig. 14. Case ACR 1: Graph showing the dramatic decrease of blood pressure after radiosurgery (arrow) and the rate of the disappearance of the acromegaly

The patient's condition was unchanged during the succeeding years but when he was readmitted for examination in the Autumn of 1976 the visual fields were found to be completely normal and the visual acuity of the left eye had increased. On the other hand, the GH values were now considerably increased. Air encephalography somewhat later showed a pronounced shrinkage of the suprasellar tumour (Fig. 15 b). These findings, combined with the patients impaired endocrine state gave further support to the idea that only the intrasellar tumour part was responsible for the acromegaly. This area will soon be given additional irradiation.

Conclusions

In patients with Cushing's disease, Nelson's syndrome, acromegaly and hyperprolactinemia, suspected to harbour a "microadenoma" of the anterior pituitary lobe, complete cure can be expected without concomitant pituitary insufficiency after treatment by stereotactic radiosurgery. Suitable for this treatment are all microadenomas detectable by discrete changes on plain

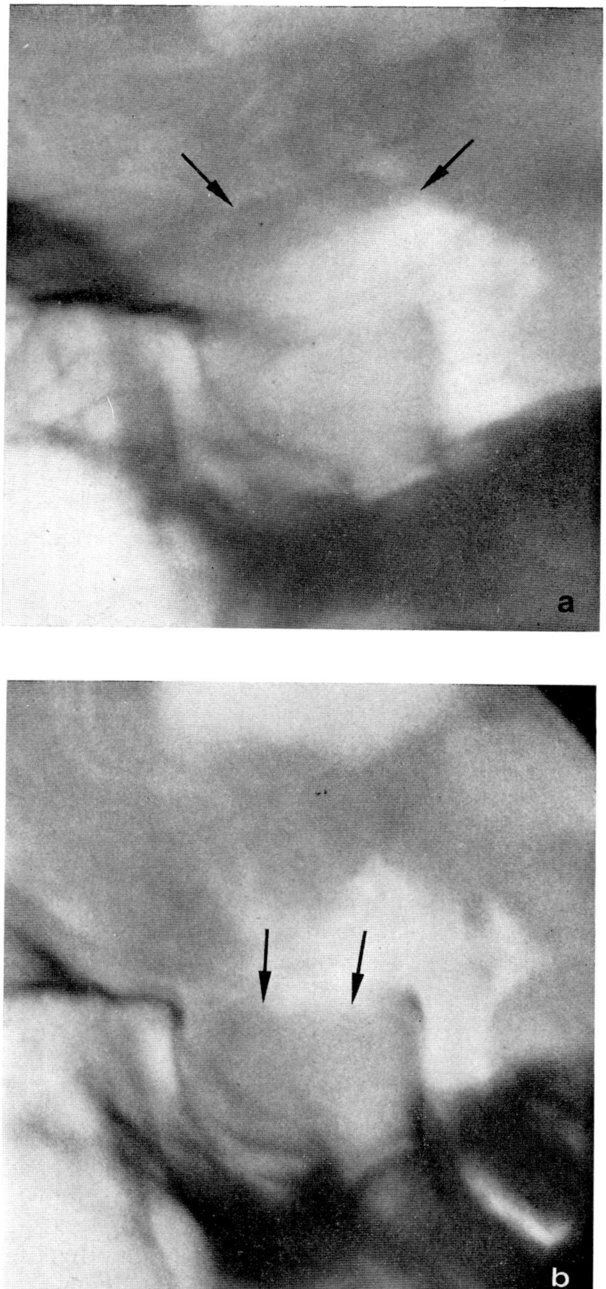

Fig. 15 a and b. Case ACR 6: Air encephalography a) before and b) six years after radiosurgery

sella x-ray and those of a size not exceeding approximately one cm in diameter. The results after radiosurgery are comparable to those of trans-sphenoidal selective adenomectomy. As it does not have the risk of complications inseparable from all open surgery, radiosurgery aims to replace open selective adenomectomy.

Arteriovenous Malformations (AVM)

In 1969, Johnson emphasized the value of radiotherapy in cases of inoperable AVM. Occasional successful cases had been reported previously (Svien and Peserico 1960, *e.g.*), but in general, irradiation was not considered a therapeutic alternative to surgery.

Encouraged by the reports mentioned, we attempted radiosurgery in an AVM case for the first time in 1970. We considered as further support in this attempt the general concept in radiobiology, that blood vessels are easily injured by ionizing radiation (cf. Rubin and Casarett 1968).

In our pilot case a sharply focused single dose of 50 Gy was administered to the feeding arteries. These vessels were initially not influenced by the irradiation but eventually they became obliterated and the AVM could no longer be visualized by angiography 19 months after treatment (Steiner *et al.* 1972). In three additional cases, each treated in a similar way with irradiation of the feeding arteries only, it was however not possible to reproduce the results of this first spectacular case. In a fourth case in which the whole AVM happened to be small enough to be covered by the radiation, angiography one year later showed no contrast filling of the AVM proper (Steiner *et al.* 1974).

In 1856, Virchow established the conditions for initiation of a thrombus, and this concept is still valid, although somewhat modified (cf. Jörgensen 1973). The following factors are mentioned as important for thrombus formation:

1. endothelial injury,
2. changes of coagulation mechanisms,
3. deviation from normal blood flow.

Since the hemodynamics of the AVM's small shunting vessels must involve abnormal blood flow, it seems reasonable that thrombus formation could be induced if the endothelium of these vessels is injuried by radiation. An adjuvant effect could possibly be obtained if antithrombolytic agents are also given, or if the coagulation mechanism is artificially activated.

The reaction to noxious radiation seems to vary with vascular size, the smallest being the most sensitive. This gives further support to the idea of irradiating preferentially the abovementioned shunting vessels. This is also in agreement with findings in animal experiments in which the basilar artery in the cat has been irradiated. These show that the small vessels of the neighbouring brain stem thrombose, whereas the basilar artery itself remains patent, in spite of being severely damaged (Nilsson *et al.* 1978).

After the pilot series, the subsequent cases were treated according to the following hypothesis:

The arterial supply of each AVM is composed of a number of "vascular units" (Fig. 16), each of which consists of one main feeder and its corresponding shunting capillary "compartment". This general arrangement can be seen in the clinical neuroradiologic studies. The anatomy of the venous outflow, on the other hand, may vary considerably and does not necessarily correspond anatomically to the "vascular unit" structure. In order to achieve a significant effect on the bulk of the AVM, at least one whole "compartment" has to be given a sufficient radiation dose. An optimal therapeutic situation is present when all shunting "compartments" can be covered by the radiation.

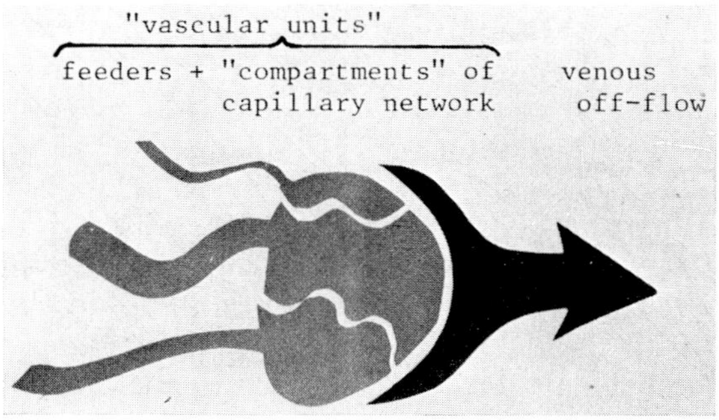

Fig. 16. Principal arrangement of the vascular components of an arteriovenous malformation

Of course, the irradiation could be directed also to one or more of the feeding arteries but even if obliteration of these could be obtained, it would be without effect unless all tributaries were "ligated". This is well known from the experience of conventional AVM surgery.

In some cases the size or shape of the AVM does not allow more than a minor part of the pathological vessels to be covered by the radiation. In these cases it is questionable whether a significant effect can be expected from radiosurgery. Nevertheless our series includes some cases belonging to this group and in most of these, radiosurgery appeared to be the only concievable treatment.

Single doses varying between 50 and 125 Gy to a target point at the centre of the vascular cluster have been used. Post-operatively a few cases have also been treated with epsilon amino caproic acid (EACA) injected intravenously for three weeks after irradiation. Whether or not this will increase the tendency for occlusion of the irradiated vessels remains to be studied.

Our experiences up to now have been reviewed recently (Backlund *et al.* 1977, Steiner *et al.* 1977) and will be summarized here.

The total number of cases treated was 35, three of which were excluded from the study because of a too short follow-up period (less than three months). The cases were grouped as follows:

A. The whole cluster of pathological vessels was covered by a sufficient dose.

B. Only a part of the cluster could be so covered.

C. Only the feeders were irradiated.

D. Only some of several feeders could be included within the radiation field.

Control angiography made about 3, 6, 12, 36 and 60 months after the treatment allowed the study of two main features:

1. Hemodynamic changes, *e.g.* diminished blood flow through the AVM and consequent narrowing of the feeding arteries and the draining veins.
2. Gradual disappearance of the pathological vessels to total obliteration.

Table 3. *AVMs Treated by Radiosurgery—Radiological Changes at Angiography 3–60 Months Postoperatively*

Results	No. of patients in Group[a]				Total
	A	B	C	D	
Total obliteration	10	—	1	—	11
Partial obliteration	1	2	1	—	4
Hemodynamic changes	2	3	—	—	5
No changes	1	6	1	4	12
Total	14	11	3	4	32

[a] For definitions, see text.

In general, if effects were registered at all, hemodynamic changes in each case have proved to be progressive in nature and most often preceeded the morphological changes. The angiographic results are compiled in Table 3. In 15 of the 32 cases obliteration was noted, though it was only partial in four of these. No changes were found in 12 cases. It must be noted, however, that some of these cases had a relatively short follow-up period. If only cases with a minimum follow-up period of seven months are studied, then 90% of the patients in Group A were cured; the remaining 10% of this group showed pronounced changes which suggest that complete obliteration will occur in the future.

In the few cases treated with EACA no evidence for an adjuvant effect has so far been noticed.

In three cases untoward effects have been observed. In one case of Group A, a left-sided occipital AVM disappeared completely, but a right-sided homonymous hemianopia appeared within three months after radiosurgery. This visual field defect is, however, of no distress to the patient.

In a 61-year old patient in Group B, a right-sided hemianaesthesia appeared 10 months after treatment. His quite extensive AVM located in the posterior part of left thalamus was subtotally obliterated after treatment. When this side-effect was noticed, a computed tomography was made which showed changes corresponding to the area irradiated, indicating a localized edema or possibly an infarction.

After this series was reported, a similar side-effect appeared six months after radiosurgery in one additional case, a young woman with a relatively large parietal AVM. Two targets separated by 17 mms were irradiated with the widest collimator to give the maximum radiation field. This may explain this patient's development of a spastic hemiparesis.

One patient in Group A bled six months after the treatment. He was from a foreign country where angiography prior to the bleeding had showed a partial disappearance of his small malformation, which had been subcortically located in the region of the right motor cortex. The intracerebral hematoma was evacuated in his home country. In an operative specimen, remnants of the AVM, a great number of vessels with organized or fresh thrombi were seen together with patent vessels (Fig. 17).

One other patient, also a foreigner, had re-bleeding 22 months after treatment. In this case, it was only possible to irradiate one of many feeding vessels, but nevertheless, angiography eight months after radiosurgery showed that the AVM had decreased in size. For practical reasons, it was impossible for the patient to return for a follow-up examination in connection with the re-bleeding.

Only one patient died in the entire group. He was the pilot case described above with total obliteration of the AVM, and he succumbed in connection with a gall bladder operation six years after radiosurgery in another hospital. Unfortunately autopsy was not performed.

The main drawback of radiosurgical treatment of AVM is the long latency period during which new haemorhages may occur. When total obliteration was achieved in the present series, it appeared 7–9 months after radiosurgery. The heavy doses used in these cases reflect an attempt at shortening this latency period. It has not been established, however, that increasing the dose correlates with an earlier radiobiological response.

Case Report I (AVM 11)

A 22-year old woman reported that at the age of 13 she had suddenly suffered from tingling in the radial part of her right hand and from a slight aphasia. The symptoms lasted only for a few days. At about the same age she had also had a second period of symptoms involving her central nervous system with insidious headaches, neck stiffness and fever, which was suspected to be a meningitis.

In September 1973, the patient suddenly felt a numbness in her right hand and right half of her face and had difficulties in speaking. Her speech was normalized gradually during the following week but the numbness in her right hand persisted. She was then examined at the neurological department with the following findings: Slight dysphasia, impaired sensation on the dorsum of her right hand and the right half of her face, and dysdiadochokinesis and slight muscular weakness in her right upper limb.

The patient was pregnant at that time, and because of this the angiographic examination was postponed until the pregnancy was terminated by Caesarean section. Angiography showed an AVM of 1.5 cm diameter, located subcortically in the central region of the left cerebral hemisphere (Fig. 18 a).

On admission to our department in April 1975 she still had paraesthesiae and numbness in her right thumb and index finger but no sensory deficit. She complained subjectively of difficulty in finding words, but the aphasia test was normal. The muscular reflexes of her right arm were slightly exaggerated. With this exception, her neurological state was normal, including neuro-ophthalmological examination.

In April 1975 the AVM was irradiated in Gamma Unit II. 100 Gy were delivered to the target point at the centre of the vascular nest. On the

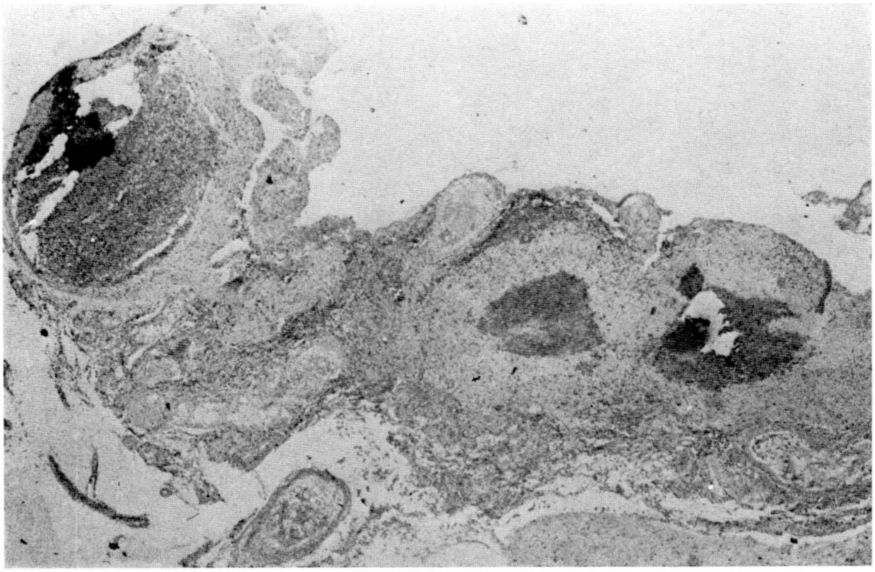

Fig. 17. Operative specimen from the region of an arteriovenous malformation which bled after radiosurgery. Thrombosed and patent vessels of various calibers are seen (Courtesy, Dr. J. H. Trumpy)

morning of the following day the patient noticed tingling and numbness in the area of her right cheek and chin for only 5–10 minutes. The symptoms from her right hand were unchanged. She returned home the day after the irradiation and was seen in the outpatient service one month later. Some days previous to this control she had noticed a sudden complete, but temporary, disappearance of the sensory symptoms of her right hand.

Control angiography was performed 4, 8, 12 and 24 months after the operation. Already at the first control the AVM was smaller and showed altered hemodynamics. Subsequent angiography showed a gradual but complete disappearance of the AVM (Fig. 18 b). Concomitantly, the patient's symptoms faded and were completely absent about one year after the treatment.

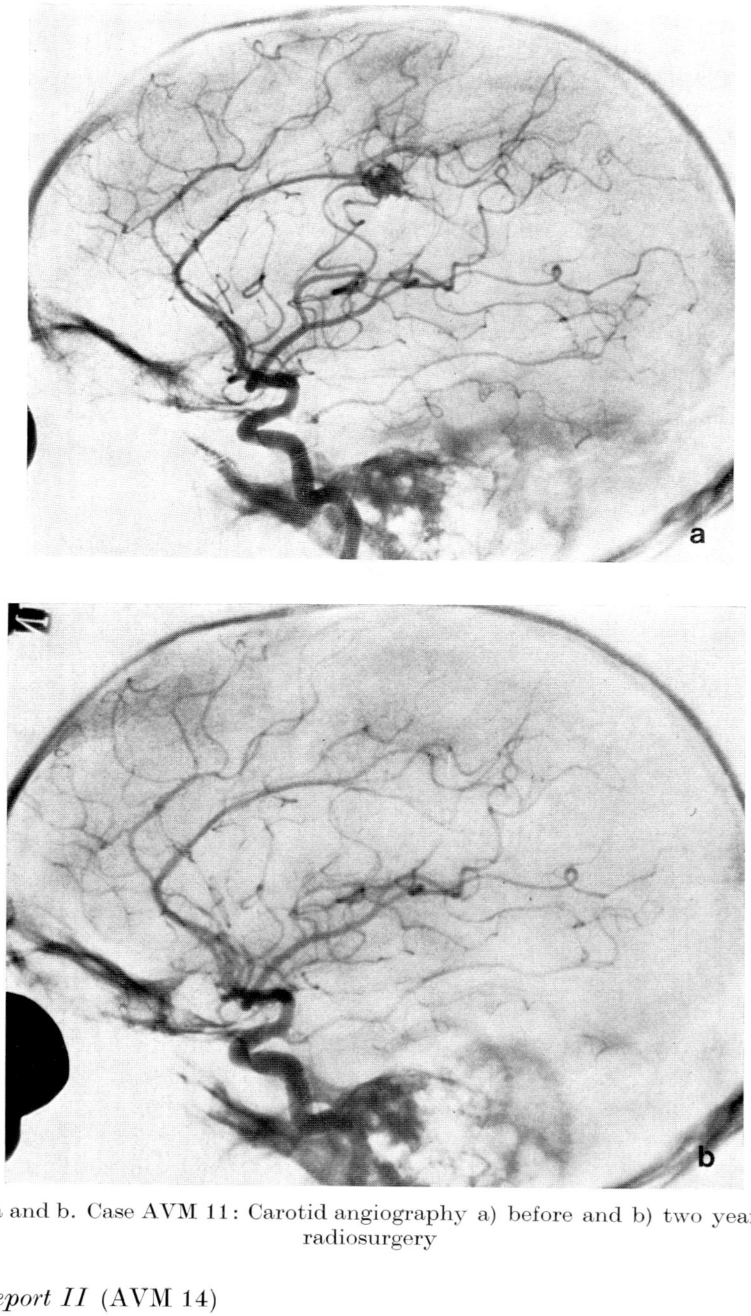

Fig. 18 a and b. Case AVM 11: Carotid angiography a) before and b) two years after radiosurgery

Case Report II (AVM 14)

A 29-year old Italian male architect was suddenly struck in 1974 by an epileptic seizure with generalized cramps. Two months later he had a second fit. He was then examined in his home country and an AVM was

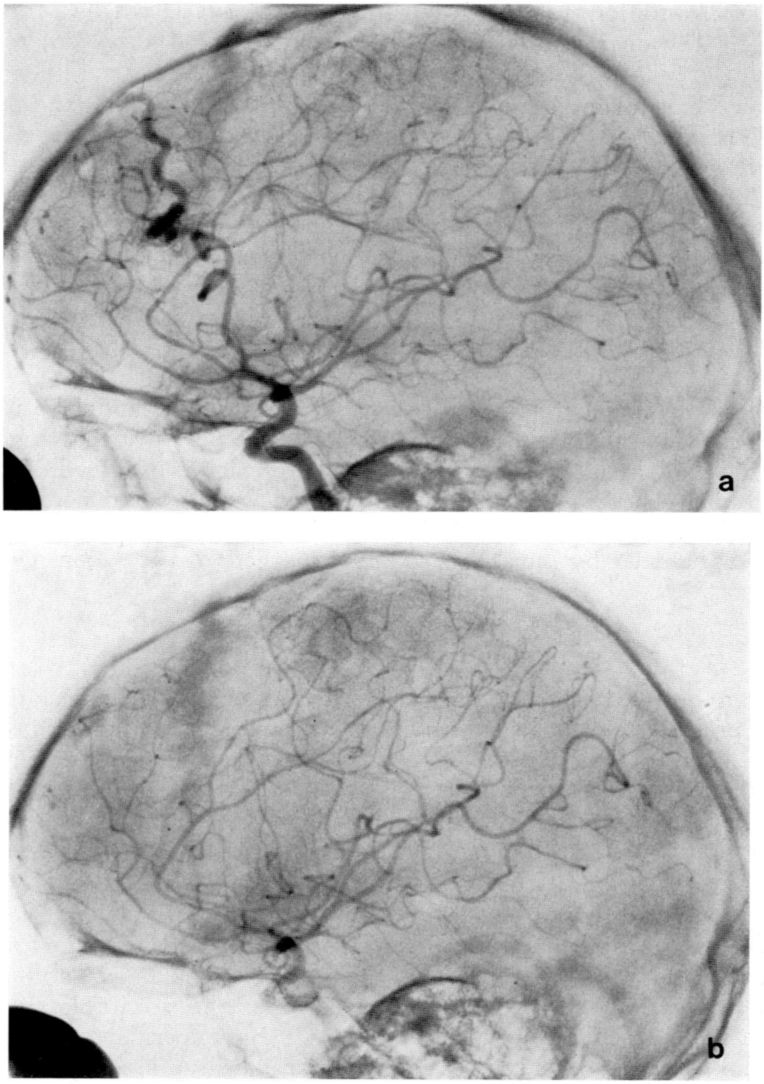

Fig. 19 a and b. Case AVM 14: Carotid angiography a) before and b) 21 months after radiosurgery

found in the right frontal region (Fig. 19 a). He was placed on anti-epileptic medication and was referred to our department for assessment.

On admission in August 1975 he presented with a normal neurologic examination. Bilateral carotid angiography revealed the AVM to be 1.5 cm in diameter and supplied by a branch from the right ascending frontal artery. As compared with previous angiography (March 1975) the width of the feeding artery had increased somewhat. The venous drainage was *via* a hypertrophic cortical vein to the superior saggittal sinus.

The malformation was irradiated in Gamma Unit II with a target dose of 75 Gy. The operative course was uneventful and the patient returned home on the following day.

The first control angiography was performed 11 months later and revealed that the diameter of the feeding artery now was of ordinary size and that the draining vein was considerably narrowed as well. Circulation through the malformation was much slower. A third angiography was performed 21 months after the operation. The malformation had now disappeared and the vasculature in that region appeared completely normal (Fig. 19 b). During the observation period the patient was well and had no seizures.

Conclusion

Stereotactic radiosurgery is a new treatment which should be used for cerebral AVMs of suitable size and location. The only drawback with this therapy is the long latency period before obliteration is obtained. Attempts at provoking the thrombosis in the irradiated vessels could possibly solve this problem. For the present, large and/or superficially located AVMs have to be treated by more conventional methods (extirpation, embolization).

General Conclusions

Any area of pathological tissue of limited extent within the skull which can be precisely outlined by x-ray or otherwise spatially defined is in principle a possible object for destruction by radiosurgery. In the future, the radiosurgical technique may possibly also be used for influencing physiological mechanisms by the delivery of sublethal doses to selected areas of tissue responsible for certain functions, *e.g.* the production of releasing factors.

Our experience during the last ten years has led to the routine use of radiosurgery in cases of hypersecreting microadenomas of the pituitary and in selected cases of craniopharyngiomas, "pinealomas" and arterio-venous malformations. For acoustic tumours, the advisable treatment program will be settled in the near future. Our experiences include also occasional cases of other inaccessible tumours such as meningiomas growing from the skull base, juvenile hypothalamic spongioblastomas, glomus jugulare tumours and retinoblastomas. In cases of non-secreting pituitary adenomas, radiosurgery has been used either as an alternative to conventional postoperative radiotherapy or as the primary treatment instead of open surgery.

The tissue of any tumour selected for radiosurgery should be microscopically classified prior to irradiation. This is easily performed by stereotactic biopsy. The author has personal experience of fine needle exploration of every conceivable region within the cranial compartment. The complication rate has been very low and does not exceed the low rate characteristic of stereotactic procedures.

A promising trend in recent years has been the application of open stereotactic techniques to common, classical neurosurgical problems. This, in combination with the experiences presented here, shows the significance of utilizing the intrinsic safety of stereotaxy in every-day neurosurgical practice.

Acknowledgements

This review has been made possible by a grant from the Swedish Cancer Society.

The clinical projects mentioned are, as a matter of course, expressions of invaluable individual contributions from many members of the Stereotactic Research Group. In preparing the present study, the following have contributed in particular:

Professor Lars Leksell, founder of radiosurgery,

Drs. Ladislau Steiner, Tiit Rähn and Georg Norén, in charge of three of the projects and

Dr. Jürgen Arndt, responsible for the radiation physics.

The author wishes to express his sincere gratitude for this cooperation.

He is further greatly indepted to Drs. Bill Chandler and Russ Anderson for valuable criticism of the text and to Miss Agneta Ringbäck for skilful secretarial assistance.

References

Arndt, J., Backlund, E.-O., Dahlin, H., Ekström, P., 1975: A computer controlled dose planning system for irradiation of small volumes of the brain with a multi cobalt unit. Proc. 3rd Congr. Soc. Radiol. Europ., Edinburgh.

Backlund, E.-O., 1969: Stereotaxic treatment of craniopharyngiomas. In Nobel Symposium 10: Disorders of the skull base region, pp. 237—244. Eds. Hamberger, C.-A., Wersäll, J. Stockholm: Almqvist & Wiksell.

Backlund, E.-O., 1973: Studies on craniopharyngiomas. III: Stereotaxic treatment with intracystic yttrium-90. Acta Chir. Scand. *139*, 237—247.

Backlund, E.-O., 1977: Treatment of craniopharyngiomas—a 10 year material, 1966—1975. Proc. 6th Int. Congr. Neurol. Surg., Sao Paulo.

Backlund, E.-O., Rähn, T., Sarby, B., de Schryver, A., Wennerstrand, J., 1972 a: Closed stereotaxic hypophysectomy by means of ^{60}Co gamma radiation. Acta Radiol. (Ther. Phys. Biol.) *11*, 545—555.

Backlund, E.-O., Johansson, L., Sarby, B., 1972 b: Studies on craniopharyngiomas. II: Treatment by stereotaxis and radiosurgery. Acta Chir. Scand. *138*, 749—759.

Backlund, E.-O., Rähn, T., Sarby, B., 1974: Treatment of pinealomas by stereotaxic radiation surgery. Acta Radiol. (Ther. Phys. Biol.) *13*, 368—376.

Backlund, E.-O., Arndt, J., Dahlin, H., Greitz, T., Leksell, L., Steiner, L., 1977: Radiosurgery in intracranial arteriovenous malformations. I: Technique. In Neurological Surgery, pp. 162—167. Eds. Carrera, R., Le Vay, D. Amsterdam-Oxford: Excerpta Medica.

Bergström, J., Greitz, T., 1976: Stereotaxic computed tomography. Amer. J. Roentgenol. *127*, 167—170.

Brismar, J., 1974: Orbital Phlebography. A method for examination of the intraorbital veins and the basal sinuses of the skull. Technique and normal anatomy Acta Radiolog. (Diagn.), Stockholm *15* (4), 369—382.

Brismar, K., Bajraktari, X., Goulatia, R., Efendić, S., 1978: The empty sella syndrome — intrasellar cisternal herniation — in "normal" patients with communicating hydrocephalus and intracranial tumours. Neuroradiology *17*, 35—43.

Dahlin, H., Rossander, K., Svedberg, J., 1970: On the selection of dose distributions in clinical cerebral radiosurgery. Proc. 9th Symposium Neuroradiologicum, Gothenburg.

Greitz, T., Backlund, E.-O., Bergström, M., Boëthius, J., Norén, G., Sundman, R., 1975: Stereotaktisk lokalisation av intrakraniella tumörer med datortomografi. Sv. Fören. f. Neuroradiol., Stockholm.

Hardy, J., Vezina, J. L., 1976: Transsphenoidal neurosurgery of intracranial neoplasm. Adv. Neurol. *15*, 261—273.

Johnson, R. T., 1969: Surgery of intracerebral haemorrhage. In Recent advances in neurology and neuropsychiatry, pp. 102—128. London: Churchill.

Jörgensen, L., 1973: Vessel wall and thrombogenesis: Vascular injury, atherosclerosis. Thrombos. Diathes. Haemorrh. (Stuttgart). Suppl. *54*, 309—316.

Kjellberg, R. N., Kliman, B., 1973: A system for therapy of pituitary tumours. In: Diagnosis and treatment of pituitary tumours, pp. 234—252. Eds. Kohler, P. O., Ross, G. T. Amsterdam: Excerpta Medica.

Kramer, S., Southard, M., Mansfield, C. M., 1968: Radiotherapy in the management of craniopharyngiomas. Amer. J. Roentgenol. *103*, 44—52.

Landolt, A. M., 1974: Can craniopharyngiomas be treated by radiotherapy? In: Progr. in pediatric neurosurgery, pp. 232—236. Eds. Bushe, K. A., Spoerri, O., Shaw, J. Stuttgart: Hippokrates.

Larsson, B., Leksell, L., Rexed, B., Sourander, P., Mair, W., Andersson, B., 1958: The high-energy proton beam as a neurosurgical tool. Nature *182*, 1222.

Lawrence, J. H., Tobias, C. A., Linfoot, J. A., Born, J. L., Chong, C. Y., 1976: Heavy particle therapy in acromegaly and Cushing's disease. J. A. M. A. *235*, 2307—2310.

Leksell, L., 1951: The stereotaxic method and radiosurgery of the brain. Acta Chir. Scand. *102*, 316—319.

Leksell, L., 1971: Stereotaxis and radiosurgery—an operative system. Springfield, Ill.: Ch. C Thomas.

Leksell, L., 1971: A note on the treatment of acoustic tumours. Acta Chir. Scand. *137*, 763—765.

Leksell, L., Herner, T., Lidén, K., 1955: Stereotaxic radiosurgery of the brain. Report of a case. Kungl. Fysiogr. Sällsk. Lund Förhandl. *25*, 1—10.

Minakova, Y. I., 1977: Personal communication.

Nilsson, A., Wennerstrand, J., Leksell, D., Backlund, E.-O., 1978: Stereotactic gamma irradiation of basilar artery in cat. A pilot study. Acta Radiol. (Oncology) *17*, 150—160.

Norén, G., Backlund, E.-O., Grepe, A., Leksell, L., 1979: Stereotactic radiosurgery in acoustic neurinomas. To be published.

Norén, G., Backlund, E.-O., 1977: Treatment of acoustic tumours by stereotactic radiosurgery. Proc. 6th Congr. Neurol. Surg., Sao Paulo.

Rubin, P., Casarett, G. W., 1968: Clinical radiation pathology, Vol. I—II. Philadelphia: W. B. Saunders.

Rähn, T., Thorén, M., Hall, K., Backlund, E.-O., 1979: Acute and short-term effects on pituitary hormone secretion after radiosurgery in patients with pituitary dependent Cushing's syndrome. To be published.

Sarby, B., Larsson, B., 1965: Fysikaliska experiment rörande förutsättningar för användning av smala gammastrålar vid cerebral strålkirurgi. Report from the Gustaf Werner Institute, Uppsala, Sweden.

Steiner, L., Leksell, L., Greitz, T., Forster, D. M. C., Backlund, E.-O., 1972: Stereotaxic radiosurgery for cerebral arteriovenous malformations. Report of a case. Acta Chir. Scand. *138*, 459—464.

Steiner, L., Leksell, L., Forster, D. M. C., Greitz, T., Backlund, E.-O., 1974: Stereotactic radiosurgery in intracranial arteriovenous malformations. Acta Neurochir. (Wien), Suppl. *21*, 195—209.

Steiner, L., Greitz, T., Leksell, L., Norén, G., Rähn, T., Backlund, E.-O., 1977: Radiosurgery in intracranial arteriovenous malformations. II: A follow-up study. In Neurological Surgery, pp. 168-180. Eds. Carrea, R., Le Vay, D. Amsterdam-Oxford: Excerpta Medica.

Svien, H. J., Peserico, J., 1960: Regression in size of arteriovenous anomaly. J. Neurosurg. *17*, 493—496.

Thorén, M., Rähn, T., Hall, K., Backlund, E.-O., 1978: Treatment of pituitary dependent Cushing's syndrome with closed stereotactic radiosurgery by means of ^{60}Co gamma radiation. Acta Endocrinol. *88*, 7—17.

Infection in Neurosurgery

J. Klastersky, L. Kahan-Coppens, and J. Brihaye

Service de Médecine Interne et Laboratoire d'Investigation Clinique H. J. Tagnon, Institut Jules Bordet; et Clinique Neurochirurgicale; Université Libre de Bruxelles, Brussels (Belgium)

Contents

There is currently a spectrum ranging from 0.5% to 10% incidence of infection in the neurosurgical literature. In a recent retrospective study it has been found that the incidence of infection for neurosurgical patients was 7.4% in the urinary tract, 2.2% in neurosurgical wounds, 2.1% in respiratory system and 1.08% miscellaneous[1].

Although neurosurgery provides the best treatment for several types of infection of the central nervous system, the present review will deal basically with the problem of infection as a consequence of a neurosurgical procedure. This aspect is important since infection following neurosurgical operations is associated with a significant morbidity and mortality and increased costs from prolonged length of hospitalization.

Clearly, infections of the central nervous system are more often the consequence of neurosurgery than infections arising in other parts of the body. However, even certain extra-neurologic hospital infections occurring in neurosurgical patients present characteristics which are directly related to the neurological status of the patient and to the type of neurosurgical procedure. Therefore, these infections will also be discussed here in order to try and offer a complete picture of the problem of sepsis in neurosurgical patients.

The microbiological features of the infections complicating neurosurgery are also somewhat different from those occurring in patients without neurosurgical lesions and thus, deserve special analysis. However, these aspects cannot be isolated from the clinical features and will not be discussed separately.

Meningitis

Meningitis occurs in neurosurgical patients in 3 main circumstances.

Firstly it may appear as a complication of a traumatic or surgical fistula of cerebrospinal fluid. Rhinorrhea and to a lesser degree otorrhea are the conditions which predispose to that complication. Usually, the meningitis is caused by *Str. pneumoniae* (pneumococcus) but other microorganisms may be involved as well. Most of these meningitides appear within days or weeks after the appearance of the fistula but occasionally they may manifest themselves after very prolonged intervals. Recurrent meningitis, sometimes over periods of years, may follow a cerebrospinal fluid fistula which may be very occasional or even not obvious at all from the clinical point of view[2]. When the cerebrospinal fluid fistula is clinically apparent, it should be corrected surgically before the possible onset of meningitis. The question arises whether patients with such cerebrospinal fluid fistulas should be treated prophylactically with penicillin or other antibiotics as long as the cerebrospinal fluid leak is present. No clear answer to this question is available in the literature; uncontrolled studies suggest that such prophylaxis is probably not effective[3]. Recently, in a controlled study we have been unable to detect any significant effect from prophylaxis with penicillin in patients with rhinorrhea or otorrhea[4]. However, it might be indicated to give antibiotics to patients who are undergoing surgery for cerebrospinal fluid fistulas on the operative day and for a few days afterwards. The selection of antibiotics to be used should be based on cultures of the nasal secretions obtained by swabbing the nasal mucosa and the nasopharynx prior to the operation and on the predictible diffusion of that antibiotic in the C.S.F. Only controlled studies can determine however whether such therapy is really useful.

Another feature which predisposes to bacterial meningitis in neurosurgical patients is the cerebrospinal fluid shunt. Shunt infection occurred in 27% of 289 hydrocephalic patients who had cerebrospinal fluid shunts inserted; the rate of infection did not vary with the type of shunt in this recent large series[5]. Most of these meningitides are caused by *Staph. epidermidis* and to a lesser degree by *Staph. aureus*; anaerobic microorganisms, such as Propionibacterium species, have also been reported as a cause of shunt infection. Infection related to cerebrospinal fluid shunts may be associated with little evidence of inflammation within the cerebrospinal fluid or systemically. The possibility of shunt infection must always be considered in febrile patients having had this type of surgery, particularly as the infection can be considerably delayed.

Cultures of the cerebrospinal fluid, especially if obtained from the shunt itself usually provide the correct diagnosis. Removal of the infected shunt in conjunction with administration of systemic antibiotics is the effective therapy. Use of systemic antibiotics alone is generally ineffective and may be associated with an increased mortality rate.

It is likely that the infecting microorganisms are introduced during the perioperative period. The possibility that prophylactic antibiotics or different shunt material might reduce the infection rate requires further study.

Shunt infections may be associated with immune complex disease, especially glomerulonephritis, similar to that seen as a complication of subacute bacterial endocarditis.

Therapy of staphylococcal meningitis should be based on *in vitro* sensitivity studies of the isolated microorganism. Penicillin-sensitive isolates can be treated with high doses of penicillin G. Most penicillin-resistant staphylococci are sensitive to methicillin. Because of the relatively low binding of methicillin to serum protein, it might be the best semi-synthetic penicillin for the treatment of staphylococcal infections of the central nervous system. No extensive data exist about the effectiveness of isoxazolyl-penicillins (oxacillin, cloxacillin) in staphylococcal meningitis. These antibiotics are heavily bound to plasma proteins and do not readily cross the blood brain barrier, at least when the meninges are not inflamed.

Chloramphenicol and cephalosporins have been unreliable agents for the treatment of staphylococcal meningitis in our experience. Vancomycin is an effective antistaphylococcal drug which is said to penetrate adequately into the cerebrospinal fluid[6]; further studies are indicated to delineate its role in the management of staphylococcal infections of the central nervous system and to assess whether it should be used intrathecally as well as by intravenous injection. The role of intrathecally injected aminoglycosides deserves also more investigation in this type of infection.

Diagnostic or surgical procedures involving the neuraxis or adjacent structures preceded the development of meningitis in 10 of 18 patients who developed nosocomial meningitis over a 25 year period in an american hospital. These hospital infections which appeared as a result of neurosurgery represented 3% of all the meningitides seen at that center during the study[7]. Occasionally, aseptic meningitis following diagnostic or surgical procedures on the central nervous system has been reported; for example, a syndrome of aseptic meningitis following posterior fossa surgery in children has been described. This form of meningitis does not respond to antibiotics but steroids in suitable doses will modify or suppress the clinical and cerebrospinal fluid picture[8]. Of course, infection or hemorhage must be ruled out before considering the diagnosis of aseptic (post-surgery) meningitis.

The majority of cases of nosocomial meningitides in neurosurgical patients are caused by *Ps. aeruginosa* and enteric gram negative bacilli. The prognosis of this type of gram negative bacillary meningitis is usually poor: depressed host defenses, multiple surgical procedures, foreign bodies and pathogenicity of infecting bacteria all contribute to a low survival rate associated with these infections. Early therapy with antibiotics which achieve adequate cerebrospinal fluid levels would appear to be necessary to minimize neurological damage and improve survival[9, 10].

Treatment of gram negative bacillary meningitis is complicated by the frequent resistance of the infecting organisms to multiple antimicrobial agents and by the failure of most chemotherapeutic agents, to enter reliably the cerebrospinal fluid.

When the offending gram negative organism is sensitive to chloramphenicol it has been our practice to treat our patients with chloramphenicol (100 mg/kg) as recommended by Rahal[11]. Chloramphenicol can also be prescribed while awaiting identification of the offending pathogen and its sensitivity to antibiotics. In our recent experience, many pathogens responsible for meningitis in neurosurgical patients have been found resistant to chloramphenicol. Therefore, now we start more often therapy with systemic and intrathecal aminoglycosides. We do not rely on other antibiotics (ampicillin, cpehalosporins, carbenicillin, etc. . . .) administered alone for the treatment of gram negative meningitis associated with neurosurgical predures; if the offending pathogen is resistant to chloramphenicol, aminoglycosides should be prescribed.

Intrathecal Administration of Antibiotics

However even in patients with inflamed meninges aminoglycosides are generally not detectable within the cerebrospinal fluid; this is in accordance with the observation that survival of neonates with gram negative meningitis correlates specifically with the sensitivity of their isolates to ampicillin which was administered concurrently. Therefore, it may be considered that for treatment of meningitis intramuscular administration of aminoglycosides cannot be consistently relied upon to give spinal fluid concentrations that exceed the minimum inhibitory concentrations required for many sensitive pathogens.

A large series of patients with meningitis due to gram negative enteric bacilli has been reported by Rahal and co-workers[12]. Sixteen of these patients were given 3 to 12 doses of 4 mg of gentamicin intrathecally in conjunction with intramuscular therapy; this regimen yielded therapeutic concentrations in the cerebrospinal fluid for 12 or 18 hours (19- to 46 μg/ml during the first 8 hours), but afterwards, the levels of gentamicin in the spinal fluid were lower than 3 μg/ml in spite of the continuation of the intramuscular injections. Favorable clinical results with intrathecal gentamicin in gram negative meningitis have been reported recently by Mangi and co-workers[13]. A sterile cerebrospinal fluid was achieved in 21/22 (95%) episodes of documented gram negative bacillary meningitis. Seventy seven percent of these patients survived their infection. However, the administration of 4 mg of gentamicin intrathecally does not sterilize the cerebrospinal fluid in some cases. Therefore a higher dosage for intrathecal gentamicin has been proposed: 8 mg given intrathecally every 24 hours (J. J. Rahal, M. S. Simberkoff, E. Rubinstein — New Engl. J. Med., letter to the editor, 291, 533, 1974) or even much higher doses: 0.5 mg/kg daily, which has been proposed by Mariel and co-workers[14]. In the latter series, levels above 20 μg/ml were maintained in the spinal fluid without any accumulation of gentamicin in spite of repeated injections and with no side-effects. However,

other investigators reported the occurrence of severe radiculitis after the administration of such high doses of gentamicin into the spinal fluid (P. Noël, H. Bondue, J. Sternon—Nouv. Presse Med., letter to the editor, 4, 196, 1975). There is no evidence that a massive increase in the dose of intrathecally administered gentamicin will be correspondingly more effective in eradicating the infection in all patients. Persistent ventriculitis has been implicated as the cause of treatment failure in several cases of neonatal meningitis[15]. Favorable outcomes resulted from intraventricular gentamicin (2 to 8 mg daily) and survival has been related to ventricular gentamicin levels of 30 μg/ml or higher. Ventriculitis may thus account for accasional treatment failures despite bactericidal antibiotic in lumbar cerebrospinal fluid. Studies in man after lumbar injection of labelled markers have shown considerable activity remaining in the same area after 24 hours. When the marker was injected in a volume exceeding 10 per cent of that of the estimated cerebrospinal fluid a high level of activity reached the basal cisterns in 1 hour. Similar studies in monkeys failed to demonstrate any diffusion of intrathecally administered substances beyond the basal cisterns unless the volume injected was at least one fourth of that of the cerebrospinal fluid[16]. High cisternal concentrations of intrathecally injected substances can be achieved, in animals, by the injection of a hyperbaric solution (10% dextrose in water) and by placing the subject in the Trendelenburg position thereafter. This technique may prove useful in treatment of meningitis in man.

Adequate ventricular levels of antibiotics can only be achieved, however, by direct intraventricular injections. Administration of 5 to 10 mg of aminoglycoside (gentamicin or tobramycin) into the lumbar intrathecal space results in levels of 27–81 μg/ml in the lumbar spinal fluid and 0–2.1 μg/ml in the ventricular fluid. By contrast, these aminoglycosides when administered directly into the cerebral ventricles produce concentrations in the lumbar fluid of 11–27 μg/ml and in the ventricular fluid of 13–40 μg/ml. All six cases treated via the ventricular route resulted in a bacteriologic cure as reported in a recent study by Kaiser and McGee[17]. Intraventricular administration of aminoglycosides thus offers a reliable means of achieving high antibiotic concentrations throughout the subarachnoid space. In adults, the neurosurgical procedure necessary to insert the reservoir or to inject the drug might occasionally have a life saving effect by decreasing the intracranial hypertension. Subcutaneous cerebrospinal fluid reservoirs have been used to treat gram negative bacillary and fungal meningitis; however, in adults at least, a high incidence of complications was reported, necessitating the removal of the reservoir or preventing the later use of intrathecal therapy. In some patients, these problems may have been a contributing cause of death or of neurological deterioration. Advantages of this mode of therapy must be carefully weighed against potential risks.

At present, intraventricular therapy has been reserved for patients who are moribund or whose therapy with parenteral plus intralumbar aminoglycosides have resulted in failure or relapse. However, it seems to us that early ventricular aspiration and intraventricular injection of antibiotics might be a decisive step in the therapy of bacterial meningitis in neurosurgical patients and should not be delayed excessively.

A provisional approach to the therapy of gram negative bacillary meningitis is summarized in Table 1. It can be seen that we still recommend a combination of intrathecal therapy and systemic administration of the aminoglycoside, combined when indicated, with a penicillin (ampicillin or carbenicillin) or a cephalosporin active against the offending microorganism, especially when synergism in vitro can be demonstrated between the

Table 1. *Provisional Approach to the Therapy of Gram Negative Bacillary Meningitis* *

Pathogen sensitive to chloramphenicol	Chloramphenicol 100 mg/kg/day systemically
Initial therapy in patients who are not moribund Organisms resistant to chloramphenicol Failure or relapse after chloramphenicol	Gentamicin or tobramycin (5 mg/kg/day) or amikacin (20 mg/kg/day) systemically, associated with a potentially synergistic penicillin or cephalosporin ** *plus intralumbar* 10 mg gentamicin or tobramycin or 20 mg amikacin every 24 hours ***
Initial therapy in moribund patients Failure or relapse after systemic plus intralumbar aminoglycoside	As above, but aminoglycosides should be given *intraventricularly*

* Adapted from Kaiser and McGee.

** See text.

*** To be administered in hyperbaric solution (10% dextrose in water); the patient is placed in the Trendelenburg position after the injection for 20 minutes.

aminoglycoside and the other drug. The importance of the synergism which can be demonstrated in vitro in the outcome of severe gram negative infection has been shown in clinical studies from this laboratory[18]. The systemic therapy in patients with meningitis is planned to eradicate extra neurologic foci of infection; but in addition some antimicrobial activity may appear in the spinal fluid from the systemic administration of highly synergistic combinations.

Brain Abscess

Head injury and surgery are responsible for approximately 20% of brain abcesses in most recent series [19, 20]. Metastatic brain abscesses and those arising from otic or paranasal sinus infections are caused by multiple microorganisms among which anaerobes are often present. Post-surgical and post-traumatic brain abscesses are more commonly due to staphylococci and gram negative bacilli. It appears that the greatest danger to the patient with a brain abscess is not the infection but the mass effect of the abscess. Patients with suspected brain abscess should undergo brain scan, computerized tomography and cerebral arteriography as the diagnostic and localizing tests of choice. Lumbar puncture is hazardous and yields no specific information. A combination of wide spectrum antibiotic therapy and surgical excision of the abscess yields results superior to other methods of treatment.

We recommend, as antibiotic therapy, chloramphenicol in high dosage (100 mg/kg). Others use a combination of penicillin plus tetracycline or chloramphenicol. Combinations of bactericidal drugs such as penicillin with bacteriostatics (tetracycline, chloramphenicol) have been shown to be antagonistic *in vitro*. The significance of such antagonism is still uncertain, but the possibility exists that it may affect unfavorably the clinical course. We do not recommend therefore the simultaneous use of penicillin with either tetracycline or chloramphenicol. This latter regimen, however, has been shown to be capable of eradicating, without surgery, intracranial suppurative disease when therapy is started early enough[21].

In addition to antibiotic therapy, various methods of treatment are still under discussion. Important differences in mortality between patients who were treated by repeated aspiration or drainage and those who were managed by operative excision of the abscess can be observed: the percentages are respectively 61%, 50% and 13%. Our personal experience is confirmatory[22]. Complete excision of the abscess is thus the most advisable method of treatment, but the choice of treatment remains closely dependent on the stage of evolution of the lesion (acute, subacute or chronic stage). Even, if in a few cases a nonencapsulated abscess can be removed by suction in the face of clinical worsening, the procedure of choice appears to be the radical enucleation of the abscess in the subacute or chronic stages, the patient having been under cover of medical treatment and sometimes after repeated aspiration or drainage. The preoperative use of steroids is still disputed and can be hazardous. However, if the perilesional oedema is life-threatening, we are of the opinion that glucocorticoids associated with antibiotics can be effective.

Long-delayed brain abscess due to retained foreign bodies are infrequent but may appear as long as 30 years after the trauma. Whatever the cause of delayed development of the abscess, a latent or a new infection, the fact that long-delayed infection occurs, must incite the surgeon to prompt debridment of the wound and to adequate antibiotic treatment.

The question whether prophylactic treatment with antibiotics would prevent intracranial infection such as meningitis or brain abscess following open trauma to the head has not been adequately answered up to now. From experience with war wounds, it appears that the main requirement in the successful treatment of these cases is attention to the wound. Prophylactically, every effort should be made at the first operation to remove all bone chips and necrotic tissue and the aim should be complete closure of the wound without drainage. It seems that cerebral tissue possesses a natural resistance to many organisms. However in the presence of a wound opening into the main cerebrospinal fluid pathways, particularly the ventricle, when foreign bodies are retained or necrotic material remains to any extent next to or within these pathways, meningitis may arise. These complicated cases might possibly benefit from systemic antiboitics along with careful surgical debridement and cleansing of the wound. High doses of penicillin G or chloramphenicol may be indicated under these circumstances[23]. However, no demonstration of definite benefit from such antimicrobial prophylaxis has yet been obtained. We have seen meningitis developing in patients with retained intraventricular foreign bodies in spite of prophylactic treatment with antibiotics to which the offending pathogen was sensitive *in vitro*.

Subdural empyema is a relatively frequent central nervous system infection, comprising one quarter of all localized intracranial bacterial infections. Subdural empyema may present with the same signs as brain abscess or/and bacterial meningitis. It may be complicated by septic venous thrombosis which leads in some cases to infarction and brain abscess. Cerebral arteriography, isotopic scanning and computerized tomography establish the diagnosis and define the location and extent of the empyema. Lumbar puncture may be followed by transtentorial herniation and should be avoided.

About 25% of these empyemas are the result of intracranial surgery. Mortality from subdural empyema remains in the range of 15%–40% and is attributed to errors in diagnosis, uncontrolled infection and delayed surgical intervention. This latter procedure is the corner stone of therapy; any delay before surgical drainage is associated with a considerable increase in morbidity and mortality[24].

Antimicrobial therapy must be discussed in relation to the expected pathogens. Most subdural empyemas following neurosurgery are caused by staphylococci and enteric gram negative bacilli. The choice of antibiotics should be influenced by *in vitro* sensitivity studies along the same lines as for bacterial meningitis.

In addition to systemic therapy with high doses of antibiotics, chloramphenicol may be introduced into the site of infection once the pus from the cerebral abscess or subdural empyema has been evacuated. Although there is no controlled study of the efficacy of this form of topical therapy, experience at our center suggests that it may be useful.

Osteomyelitis and Epidural Abscess

Osteomyelitis of the skull or of the spine and epidural abscesses are considered together because of their close anatomic relationship as well as their frequent simultaneous occurrence. The cause of either may be traumatic or non traumatic. Osteomyelitis of the skull and epidural abscesses are most frequently the consequence of infection from the paranasal sinuses and mastoid but may occur following craniotomy. Epidural abscess may also occur in the postoperative period without significant involvement of the skull.

Early diagnosis of osteomyelitis of the skull may be difficult because of the late appearance of radiological evidence of osteomyelitis. Clinically the inflammatory signs may be very mild. In other patients there may be generalized sepsis with headache and local tenderness; if neurological signs develop, this suggests the presence of an epidural abscess.

Vertebral osteomyelitis occurs as a consequence of septicemic infection or surgery, especially disc surgery. It may be associated with spinal epidural abscess. Indeed, 16% of epidural abscesses were postoperative infections in a recent study[25].

The progression from spinal ache to root pain to weakness followed by paralysis continues to be characteristic of spinal epidural abscess.

Although the disease is uncommon, the complications are so serious that prompt diagnosis and treatment are of paramount importance. Most cases of postoperative osteomyelitis and epidural abscesses are caused by staphylococci and, to a lesser extent, by enteric gram negative bacilli. Once again therapy must combine surgical drainage, especially if an abscess is present and antimicrobial therapy similar to that recommended for brain abscess and subdural empyema.

Disc Space Infection

Infection may occur in the disc space following laminectomy and excision of a protruded disc. The incidence is not known, but it appears to be rare. It is generally confined to the lumbar area where most ruptured discs occur. This type of infection in the disc space is one of the unrecognized causes of unsatisfactory results following disc surgery. There is usually satisfactory primary healing of the operative wound without evidence of complication or infection. The clinical picture in disc space infection tends to be fairly typical. Following an asymptomatic period, severe back pain develops. The pain is usually out of proportion to the findings on physical examination, except for severe muscle spasm. The patients do not have systemic signs of infection unless the infection has extended outside the disc space.

Radiographic changes are not seen during the first few weeks. Later, the disc space shows narrowing. The first bony changes are seen in the region of the vertebral body adjacent to the disc space. Later, there may be gross destruction of the vertebral body. Sclerosis then develops with new bone formation and fusion between the adjacent vertebral takes place[26].

Needle aspiration of the disc space rarely reveals pus but more often shows evidence of chronic inflammatory changes. Surgical intervention is not indicated unless there is evidence of systemic reaction and the possibility of peridural abscess exists. The patients should be treated with antibiotics and bed rest. Since these infections are usually caused by staphylococci, high doses of an antistaphylococcal penicillin (methicillin, oxacillin, cloxacillin) or lincomycin are indicated.

Pulmonary Infections

Pulmonary complications in neurosurgery are extremely frequent[27] and can be best prevented by a cooperative effort by both anesthetist and neurosurgeon along with an adequate policy as far as the use of antibiotics is concerned. Early intubation is to be encouraged. Regulation of ventilation and maintenance of oxygen carrying capacity are important for the healing of diseased cerebral tissue in any post-injury or post-operative patient.

Among these pulmonary complications, broncho-pulmonary infections are among the most frequent and important from their influence on morbidity and mortality. Patients with tracheostomies, especially when unconscious, and unable to collaborate with physiotherapists in securing an adequate bronchial drainage present a high frequency of broncho-pulmonary infections caused by *Ps. aeruginosa* and other gram negative enteric bacilli which are often resistant to many antibiotics outside the aminoglycosides. In our hospital, gram negative bronchopneumonias, caused by microorganisms sensitive to aminoglycosides *in vitro*, responded favorably to systemic therapy with gentamicin or a similar antibiotic (sisomicin, tobramycin, amikacin) in only 7 (26%) out of 27 patients with tracheostomy and impaired consciousness who had been admitted to a neurosurgical unit. These poor results may be due, in part at least, to the poor penetration of aminoglycosides into the bronchial secretions. This phenomenon has been documented by several investigators including ourselves[28]. In crossover studies in man, we have been able to show that the concentrations of gentamicin achieved within the bronchial secretions (less than 1 μg/ml) after the IM injection of 2 mg/kg were not adequate to inhibit most strains of Pseudomonas isolated from infected patients. Conversely, endotracheally administered gentamicin resulted in high and sustained concentrations within the bronchial secretions which were many times superior to the minimum bactericidal concentration required to inhibit 100% of the strains of *Ps. aeruginosa* in our hospital. Therefore, endotracheally administered gentamicin has been compared to intramuscularly administered gentamicin in patients with tracheostomy and serious broncho-pulmonary gram negative infections. In a randomized double blind study, 20 patients which severe bronchopneumonias caused by gram negative bacilli were treated with carbenicillin plus systemically administered sisomicin; they received in addition by the endotracheal route 25 mg of sisomicin or a placebo. Among the patients who could be evaluated, 8 received sisomicin endotracheally and 6 responded well; conversely in the placebo group, only 3 out of 8 patients responded to therapy[29]. This study suggets clearly an advantage of endotracheally administered aminoglycosides over a placebo in severe gram negative bronchopneumonias in tracheotomized patients.

The severity of gram negative bronchopneumonia superimposed on tracheostomy in neurosurgical patients prompted us also to examine the possibility of preventing this type of infection by endotracheal administration of gentamicin. We were able to show that endotracheal prophylaxis with gentamicin significantly decreases the incidence of colonization of the tracheal secretions in tracheostomized patients by gram negative bacilli and decreases the frequency of bacteriologically proved episodes of respiratory tract infections[30]. However, the bacteria isolated from gentamicin-treated patients were more resistant to gentamicin than the microorganisms recovered from the placebo-treated patients. A few highly resistant strains were isolated, in this series, from the patients who received endotracheal gentamicin and were responsible for colonization and occasionnal superinfection in other patients in the same unit. It is clear therefore that the benefits of a procedure which is capable of preventing serious and potentially fatal infections must be weighed against the risk of producing within the hospital environment pathogens highly resistant to aminoglycosides. A similar problem has been encountered by Feeley and co-workers[31] who used endobronchial prophylaxis with polymyxin B, administrated by

Table 2. *Indications for the Use of Endotracheally Administered Aminoglycosides*

Prevention of Gram negative colonisation of tracheostomized or intubated patients in intensive care units (especially if unconscious) Eradication of epidemics of nosocomial pneumonias caused by Gram negative bacilli in intensive care units	Direct endotracheal injection or aerosolization * of 40 mg of gentamicin 3 times daily
Therapy of Gram negative bronchopneumonias	Direct endotracheal injection or aerosolization * of 40 mg of gentamicin, 3 times daily, combined with systemic administration of gentamicin (80 mg 8-hourly) associated with a penicillin or a cephalosporin acting synergistically with the aminoglycoside

* Aerosols should be given only to patients who are capable of cooperating with physiotherapists; endotracheal injections are given with a plastic catheter, deeply introduced into the trachea through the tracheostomy or through a transtracheal catheter, in a volume of 5–10 ml of saline over a 5 minute period. The injections are given 3 times daily with the patient lying once in the left lateral decubitus, once in the right lateral decubitus and once in the dorsal decubitus position.

aerosol to prevent pneumonia in seriously ill patients. These investigators suggested that some form of alternating-cycle method of administration of endotracheally administered antibiotics might be necessary to take advantage of the efficacy of that technique in preventing gram negative pneumonia and simultaneously preventing the emergence of antibiotics-resistant organisms. These expectations have been partially verified in a study, performed in our hospital, in which we showed that endotracheal prophylaxis with a combination of kanamycin plus polymyxin was as effective as that using gentamicin but prevented the emergence of gentamicin-resistant strains. Another possible limitation to the use of endotracheal prophylaxis and therapy with aminoglycosides is the fear of potential toxicity resulting from systemic absorption of the locally applied aminoglycosides which may result, if systemic aminoglycosides are given at the same time, in excessive blood levels. Direct endotracheal injection of 80 mg of gentamicin produces blood concentrations of gentamicin in the range of 1 μg/ml over the 2 hours following the injection whereas aerosolization, which produces lower but still significant concentrations in the sputum, is not responsible for any significant absorption of gentamicin into the blood.

It might be useful therefore to reduce systemic doses of gentamicin and to closely monitor serum levels in order to avoid toxicity when systemic gentamicin is combined with tracheal instillation. This may be essential in patients with impaired renal function. In spite of these limitations prophylactic endotracheal administration of aminoglycosides is probably indicated to control epidemics of *Ps. aeruginosa* and other gram negative enteric bacilli infection in intensive care units and possibly indicated to protect a high-risk patient from acquiring pneumonia caused by these organisms. Whenever such prophylaxis is used there must be careful surveillance of sputum cultures and antibiotic sensitivities for rapid detection of the emergence of resistant organisms. The endotracheal administration of aminoglycosides is definitely indicated in patients with proven gram negative bacillary infection of the bronchopulmonary tract; these indications are summarized in Table 2.

It is important, at this point, to stress that excessive use of antibiotics in patients admitted to intensive care units often results in severe hospital infections caused by resistant bacteria. This has been well demonstrated by Price and Sleigh who controlled an epidemic due to a resistant strain of Klebsiella in a neurosurgical unit only by withdrawal of all antibiotics[32]. This is not to say that antimicrobial agents are useless, but it must be realized that the use of unnecessary antibiotics carries a great risk of added infection which is largely preventable by a policy of restriction of the use of antibiotics, especially of prophylactic antibiotics.

Wound Infection

There are no special rules to deal with wound infections in neurosurgical patients as compared to similar infections in other patients. Prophylaxis with antibiotics is to be discouraged with the possible exception of cases of rhinorrhea and heavily contaminated traumatic wounds. In both cases penicillin G is probably the drug of choice and should be given for a short period of time in the case of contaminated wounds and until the cerebrospinal fluid leak has stopped in patients with rhinorrhea or otorrhea. Prophylaxis with antibiotics however is no substitute for correct surgical treatment of rhinorrhea or for careful debridement of traumatic wounds.

Among wound infections, those which are associated with prolonged intravenous administration of fluids and medication deserve special mention with respect to topical therapy with antibiotics. These intravenous perfusions are the source of septicemia in about 2% of patients and thus represent a considerable hazard[33]. A few earlier studies have indicated that antibiotics (bacitracin, neomycin, polymyxin) were effective in reducing the frequency of infection associated with intravenous polyethylene catheters. Other studies, however, failed to confirm these results, suggesting rather that the prophylactic antibiotics were chiefly responsible for a change in the nature of the offending pathogens. Moreover, it has become clear that that a standardized approach to the insertion and surveillance of intravenous catheters is highly effective by itself in preventing most episodes of infection linked to their use[34].

Bacteriuria After Indwelling Catheterization

When an indwelling catheter has been in the bladder for 24 hours, the incidence of bacteriuria in patients whose urine was previously sterile is about 50%. After four days of continuous catheterization 98–100% of patients develop 100,000 or more bacteria per ml of urine. The bacteriuria that follows the use of indwelling catheters is due to the continuous entry of bacteria into the bladder when the catheter is in place. These bacteria are members of the fecal flora of the perineum. Bacteriuria resulting from urinary tract instrumentation, including indwelling bladder catheters, is the major cause of gram negative septicemia in hospitalized patients; a conservative figure for mortality in patients with gram negative septicemia is 30%. This makes obvious the need for some measures in order to prevent bacteriuria in patients with indwelling bladder catheters and its possible consequences. Systemic chemoprophylaxis is ineffective but, on the other hand, highly significant protection against the development of bacteriuria is afforded by the use of a method employing a constant rinse of the catheterized bladder with a solution possessing broad antibacterial activity[35]. A solution containing neomycin and polymyxin B can be used (stock solution of neomycin 40 mg and polymyxin 20 mg in 30 ml of saline, to be poured into 1 liter of isotonic saline which is infused over a 24 hour period). An alternative to the use of topical antibiotics is a solution with 0.25% acetic acid; it has been shown as effective as topical antibiotics in preventing bacteriuria in patients with indwelling bladder catheters.

Catheter-associated urinary tract infection remains a significant infection hazard despite available methods of prevention. Many pathogens responsible for it are transmitted between catheterized patients by passive carriage on the hands of attendants. Clustering of patients with indwelling catheters may further increase the colonization of the urinary tract arising from infected patients. Attention to these aspects may further decrease the risks associated with the use of bladder catheters.

Conclusions

It seems clear that neurosurgical procedures predispose significantly to serious infections, both within and outside the central nervous system. Among these infections, meningitis and broncho-pulmonary infections are those which require aggressive medical therapy, especially if gram negative bacilli are the offending pathogens. Thus the medical therapy to be employed in these infections has been discussed extensively and a strong recommendation has been made for the use of topical aminoglycosides, by the intrathecal and the endotracheal routes for meningitis and bronchopneumonia respectively. The other neurological infections discussed here (cerebral abscess, subdural empyema, osteomyelitis, epidural abscess) must be treated primarily by surgical drainage or excision. Antibiotics, although important, have a secondary role.

The other extra-neurological infections, beside broncho-pulmonary infections, can be adequately prevented if sufficient attention is paid to

Table 3. *Schematic Summary of Important Characteristics of Antibiotics Which are Useful for the Neurosurgical Patient*

Drug	Spectrum	C. S. F. diffusion	Adminis-tration	Dose/24 h	Interval between successive doses	
Penicillin G	Gram positive cocci (except resistant Staphylococci)	10 to 30% when meningitis present	I.V. I.M.	250,000 U.I/kg	6 h	Possible allergic reaction
Cephalosporins	Cfr. Penicillin G + gram negative bacilli* except Ps. aeruginosa	Poor: maximum 5% of serum levels when meningitis present	I.V. I.M. P.O.	50–100 mg/kg	8 h	Reduce dosage if renal impairment
Carbenicillin	Cfr. Penicillin G + gram negative bacilli except Klebsiella	20% of serum levels when meningitis present	I.V.	300–500 mg/kg	6 h	Produces hypokalaemia and brings excess of sodium (5 mEq/g) Possible allergic reaction Reduce dosage if renal impairments
Chloramphenicol	Wide spectrum including gram positive and gram negative pathogens except Ps. aeruginosa. Well active on anaerobes	30 to 50% of serum levels even without meningitis	P.O. I.V. in loco	maximum 100 mg/kg	6–8 h	Reversible pancytopenia Medullary aplasia (1/60,000)
Vancomycin	Staphylococci and enterococci	Probably poor	I.V. intrathecaly	250 mg/kg 20 mg/24 h	12 h	Ototoxicity at high serum levels Reduce dosage if renal impairment
Methicillin	Staphylococci (some strains are resistant; see in vitro tests)	10% when meningitis present	I.V.	100–400 mg/kg	4–6 h	Nephritis Possible allergic reaction
Gentamicin	Gram negative bacilli*	10–20 % when meningitis present (results in very low levels however)	I.V. I.M.	3 mg/kg	8 h	Renal toxicity (tubular) Ototoxicity Reduce dosage and increase intervals of time if renal impairment

* Excluding Hemophilus influenzae and Bacteroïdes sp.

techniques which have been recognized to be of prophylactic value against infections associated with intravenous or indwelling bladder catheters.

Generally speaking, the use of prophylactic systemic antibiotics must be discouraged; in most circumstances, its effectiveness is doubtful. Moreover there is a clear indication that the use of antibiotics, especially in small units, is associated with the emergence of antibiotic-resistant bacteria, which can turn into serious pathogens.

In conclusion, we should stress, that close clinical collaboration between neurosurgeon, anaesthetist and medical bacteriologist will result in the optimal care for neurosurgical patients, and the avoidance of the frequent infectious complications to which they are prone.

References

1. Green, J. R., Kanshepolsky, J., Turkian, B., 1974: Incidence and significance of central nervous system infection in neurosurgical patients. Advances in Neurology *6*, 223—228.
2. Levin, S., Nelson, K. E., Spies, H. W., Lepper, M. H., 1972: Pneumococcal meningitis the problem of the unseen cerebrospinal fluid leak. Amer. J. Med. Sci. *264*, 319—327.
3. MacGee, E. C., Cauthen, J. C., Brackett, C. E., 1970: Meningitis following acute traumatic cerebrospinal fluid fistula. J. Neurosurg. *33*, 312—316.
4. Klastersky, J., Sadeghy, B., Brihaye, J., 1976: Antimicrobial prophylaxis in patients with rhinorrhea or otorrhea: a double-blind study. Surg. Neurol. *6*, 111—114.
5. Schönbaum, S. C., Gardner, P., Shillito, J., 1975: Infection of serebrospinal fluid shunts: epidemiology, clinical manifestations and therapy. J. Infect. Dis. *131*, 543—552.
6. Hawley, H. B., Gump, D. W., 1973: Vancomycin therapy of bacterial meningitis. Amer. J. Dis. Child. *126*, 261—264.
7. Hodges, G. R., Perkins, R. L., 1976: Hospital associated bacterial meningitis. Amer. J. Med. Sci. *271*, 335—341.
8. Carmel, P. W., Fraser, R. A. R., Stein, B. M., 1974: Aseptic meningitis following posterior fossa surgery in children. J. Neurosurg. *41*, 44—48.
9. Mangi, R. J., Quintiliani, R., Andriole, V. T., 1975: Gram negative bacillary meningitis. Amer. J. Med. *59*, 829—836.
10. Buckwold, F. J., Hand, F., Hansenbout, R. R., 1977: Hospital acquired bacterial meningitis in neurosurgical patients. J. Neurosurg. *46*, 494—500.
11. Rahal, J. J., 1972: Treatment of gram negative bacillary meningitis in adults. Ann. Int. Med. *77*, 295—302.
12. Rahal, J. J., Hyams, P. J., Simberkoff, M. S., Rubinstein, E., 1974: Combined intrathecal and intramuscular gentamicin for gram negative meningitis. Pharmacologic study of 21 patients. New Engl. J. Med. *290*, 1394—1398.
13. Mangi, R. J., Holstein, L. L., Andriole, V. T., 1977: Treatment of gram negative bacillary meningitis with intrathecal gentamicin. Yale J. Biol. Med. *50*, 31—41.
14. Mariel, C., Veyssier, P., Pechere, J. C., 1971: Concentration de gentamicine dans le liquide céphalo-rachidien après administration par voie I.M. et par voie intrathécale lombaire. Gazette med. franç. *79*, 21—26.
15. Salmon, J. H., 1972: Ventriculitis complicating meningitis. Amer. J. Dis. Child. *124*, 35—40.
16. Rieselbach, R. E., Di Chiro, G., Freireich, E. J., 1962: Subarachnoid distribution of drugs after lumbar injection. New Engl. J. Med. *267*, 1273—1278.
17. Kaiser, A. B., McGee, Z. A., 1975: Aminoglycoside therapy of gram negative bacillary meningitis. New Engl. J. Med. *293*, 1215—1220.
18. Klastersky, J., 1976: The use of synergistic combinations of antibiotics in patients with haematological diseases. Clin. Haematol. *5*, 361—377.

19. Brewer, N. S., MacCarty, C. S., Wellman, W. E., 1976: Brain abscess: a review of recent experience. Ann. Int. Med. *82*, 571—576.
20. Samson, D. S., Clark, K., 1973: A current review of brain abscess. Amer. J. Med. *54*, 201—210.
21. Heineman, H. H., Braude, A. I., Osterholm, J. L., 1971: Intracranial suppurative disease. Early presumptive diagnosis and successful treatment without surgery. J. Amer. Med. Assoc. *218*, 1542—1547.
22. Martin, P., Brihaye, J., Martin, Ph., 1960: A propos de 53 cas d'abcès encéphaliques. Neuro-Chirurgie *6*, 299—309.
23. Hagan, R., 1971: Early complications following penetrating wounds of the brain. J. Neurosurg. *34*, 132—141.
24. Kaufman, D. M., Miller, M. H., Steigbigel, N. H., 1975: Subdural empyema: analysis of 17 recent cases and review of the literature. Medicine *54*, 485—498.
25. Baker, A. S., Ojemann, R. G., Swartz, M. N., Richardson, E. P., 1975: Spinal epidural abscess. New Eng. J. Med. *293*, 463—468.
26. Thibodeau, A. A., 1967: Closed space infection following removal of lumbar intervertebral disc. Clin. Neurosurg. *14*, 337—360.
27. Ducker, T. B., Redding, J. S., 1976: Pulmonary complications in neurosurgery. Clin. Neurosurg. *23*, 483—493.
28. Odio, W., Van Laer, E., Klastersky, J., 1975: Concentration of gentamicin in bronchial secretions after intramuscular and endotracheal administration. J. Clin. Pharmacol. *15*, 518—524.
29. Klastersky, J., Carpentier-Meunier, F., Kahan-Coppens, L., Thijs, J. P., 1978: Endotracheally administered antibiotics for gam negative bronchopneunomia. Chest (in press).
30. Klastersky, J., Huysmans, E., Weerts, D., Hensgens, C., Daneau, D., 1974: Endotracheally administred gentamicin for the prevention of infections of the respiratory tract in patients with tracheostomy; a double blind study. Chest *65*, 650—654.
31. Feeley, T. W., Du Moulin, G. C., Hedley-Whyte, J., Bushnell, L. S., Gilbert, J. P., Feingold, D. S., 1975: Aerosol polymyxin and pneumonia in seriously ill patients. New Engl. J. Med. *293*, 471—475.
32. Price, D. J. E., Sleigh, J. D., 1970: Control of infection due to Klebsiella aerogenes in a neurosurgical unit by withdrawal of all antibiotics. Lancet *2*, 1213—1215.
33. Collins, R. N., Braun, P. A., Zinner, S. H., Kass, E. H., 1968: Risk of local and systemic infection with polyethylene intravenous catheters. A prospective study of 213 catheterizations. New Engl. J. Med. *279*, 340—343.
34. Goldmann, D. A., Maki, D. G., Rhame, F. S., Kaiser, A. B., Tenney, J. H., Bennett, J. V., 1973: Guidelines for infection control in intravenous therapy. Ann. Int. Med. *79*, 848—850.
35. Martin, C. M., Bookrajian, E. N., 1962: Bacteriuria prevention after indwelling urinary catheterization. A controlled study. Arch. Int. Med. *110*, 703—711.

Spasticity—Clinical Classification and Surgical Treatment*

C. Gros

Centre Hospitalier Universitaire, Montpellier (France)

With 13 Figures

Contents

* Problems of neurogenic bladder will not be studied in this article. Cf.: Pedersen, E. Acta neurol. Scand. Suppl. 20, Vol. 42 (1966), 184 p.

Keywords: Functional Electric Stimulation FES, Myelotomy, Neurotomy, Radicotomy, Spasticity, SP.

I. Introduction

A better understanding of spasticity and of its pathophysiology has progressively emerged from the period of pure neurological description. Spasticity should no longer be considered either as unavoidable during the recovery of a motor deficit, or as an irreversible state.

Early diagnosis and treatment of perinatal CNS injuries, early and permanent nursing of hemiplegic or paraplegic patients would prevent or reduce spasticity. So, identical CNS lesions may follow different routes of rehabilitation, depending on the therapy.

This supposes that, beside the notion of cybernetic regulation, there must exist a more flexible pathophysiology of the CNS and specially of the cord.

Segmental and suprasegmental control of alpha and gamma motoneuron activity are dependant on the pool of interneurons, which work as the main regulation system of motor tone.

Any surgical lesion which reduces facilitating influences on alpha motoneurons, reduces spasticity in greater or less degree. Any physiological stimulation that corrects unbalanced muscular tone, would be beneficial.

All these treatments are effective through their action on the interneuron pool.

This is the common "denominator" of all apparently unconnected treatments, like neurotomies, peripheral electric stimulations, posterior radiculotomies, myelotomies and so forth.

When to operate and what must be done is the first and more difficult problem. This is dependant on careful clinical control of every case, by an interdisciplinary team where physical therapists and neurosurgeons work together.

This is the only way to achieve a clear continuing view of what is useful and what is handicapping in every case of spasticity, with possible treatment in mind.

Specific treatment must be varied according to the pattern of spasticity.

The theoretical basis, surgical technique, results of electrical stimulation, neurotomies, posterior radiculotomies, myelotomies, etc. . . . are presented with their indications.

Spasticity is the pathological state of a patient who suffers from increased and uncontrolled tone. The word tonus was first used by Mueller in 1838 and since that time has remained controversial.

Initially described as the "muscular tension at rest", its reflex nature was demonstrated by Brondgeest in 1860; it has been shown to require the integrity of the dorsal roots[10].

Hughes Bennett[5] in 1888 described "some muscular hypertonicity in paralysis" which stresses the relationship between decreased power and increased muscular tension. This was simultaneously described by Charcot as "rigidité élastique et plastique" and by Babinski under the term of "contractures tendino- et cutanéo-réflexes".

All these definitions cover a wide field in clinical neurology which we will now refer to as "spasticity". The word spasticity must be understood as including not only increased muscular tonus, but also increased tendon reflexes, Babinski sign, paroxysmal contractures and musculo-tendinous contracture.

Increased muscular tone is usually associated with pyramidal tract lesions; the word spasticity is reserved for disorders wherein it is the major feature of the clinical picture.

Neurosurgical treatment of spasticity must be considered as the first step in functional neurosurgery with the posterior rhizotomies of O. Foerster in 1908[28]; the way is still open for new neurophysiological research and surgical procedures.

II. Pathophysiology

Understanding of the problems of spasticity progressed through experimental research in animals and anatomo-clinical observations made in man. In 1898, Sherrington[99] repeated mesencephalic transection in the cat, an experiment originally done by Brondgeest. The state of decerebrate rigidity thus produced, is present at rest, is increased by passive displacement if rapid, and involves particularly the antigravity muscles.

This rigidity disappears after section of the posterior roots, thus it appears to be an exaggeration of a proprioceptive reflex with the receptor organ in the muscle itself. This was confirmed by Liljestrand and Magnus[66] who obtained reduction in decerebrate rigidity in the cat's triceps by an injection of Procaine into the muscle, without removing the response to motor stimulation. Walshe[124] successfully used this method to reduce rigidity in patients who presented with spastic hemiplegia.

The selective effect of Procaine infiltration on spasticity can be explained by the presence of sensitive small fibers (gamma fibers) which innervate the muscle spindles. Thus one is able to speak of a gamma spasticity.

Since the work of Sherrington, another type of spasticity has been produced by Pollock and Davis[88] which follows the ligature of the carotid and vertebral arteries; this rigidity is not removed by posterior radicotomy, but only by Procaine block of large motor fibers and has been called alpha spasticity.

Thus two types of spasticity are recognized, those which are due to an exaggeration of proprioceptive reflexes, gamma spasticity, and those which are due to an isolated alpha hyperactivity.

By injection into the sciatic nerve of spastic patients, G. Rushworth[98] has confirmed in man that Procaine reduces spasticity without affecting motor function.

He says "Many spastic states depend on the integrity of gamma motor fibers to the muscle spindles . . . Because it is probable that in spasticity an increased gamma motoneuron discharge causes a hyperexcitability of the annulo-spinal ending and thus an increased response of the muscle to stretch".

Neuro-physiological mechanisms which are brought to play in spasticity can be better understood when one takes into account the actual knowledge that exists of the alpha motoneuron and its segmental, inter-segmental and supra-segmental control (J. Cadilhac[12]).

The integrity of the alpha motoneuron is as necessary for phasic contrac tion as for tonic muscular contraction. Granit[37] and Eccles[24, 25, 26] have established the reasons for this duality by characterizing the alpha motoneurons which control tone, as large rapidly conducting fibers and motoneurons that are concerned with alpha phasic functions, as small fibers with a rapid emission (type I a and type I b according to Lloyd' classification).

Hyperexcitability in the first system explains spasticity . . . disturbances of motor function being dependant on phasic motoneurons.

1. The Segmentary Control of Alpha Motoneurons

The stretch reflex of Sherrington or myotatic reflex, explains how a muscle regulates its tension by reason of the degree of stretch to which it is subjected. The stretch reflex receptor is made up of the neuro-muscular spindle, which is stimulated by the elongation of the muscle and transmits its information by type I a fibers, large caliber fibers with a rapid propagation speed, to the alpha motoneuron. The investigation of the motor response to tendinous or electrical stimulation, constituting the monosynaptic reflex of Hoffmann, permits investigation of eventual modifications to the stretch reflex.

This reflex is influenced both by afferent sensory impulses and by impulses transmitted by the gamma system.

Extra-fusorial sensory afferent impulses (the tendinous organs of Golgi, cutaneous receptors) have a facilitating or inhibitory effect on the alpha motoneuron. The Golgi's organs via the type I b fibers have an opposing action to those of the fusorial receptors; given a certain degree of stretch they cause a brisk release of resistance (the Clasp-Knife phenomenon) by reason of their dominant action on the myotatic effect.

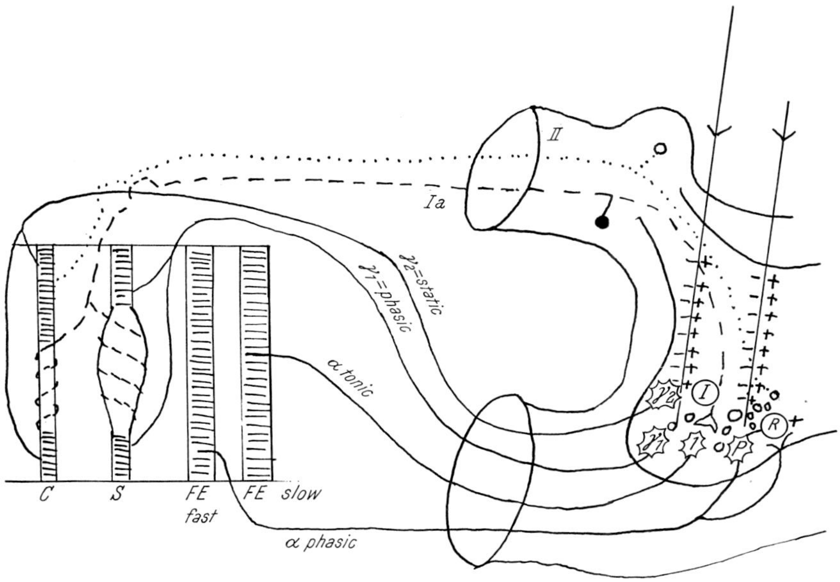

Fig. 1. Segmental level control of tonus (after Tardieu). *C* Chain fiber, *S* bag fiber, *FE* extra fusorial fiber, *T* tonic α motoneuron, *R* Renshaw cells, *P* phasic α motoneuron, γ presynaptic inhibiting interneuron, γ_1 fuso motor fibers coming to "bag", 0_2 fuso motor fibers coming to "chain", + and — supramedullary inhibiting influences (+), facilitating influence (—) on α and γ motoneurons

Stimulation of exteroceptive receptors causes the release of the defensive reflexes, the triple retreat. They also appear to have a presynaptic inhibitory effect (Lundberg[67]).

Gamma motoneuron innervation of the muscular bundle assures the maintenance of permanent tension; we have seen that this state of tension located in the spindle is transmitted by I a and II fibers to the alpha motoneuron.

Studies of the gamma motoneuron have permitted the description of fibers of different sizes with individual functions, for example those concerned with the regulation of posture (dynamic gamma fibers) others in tonic balance movement (static gamma fibers) (Fig. 1).

In spasticity there is a hyperactivity of the dynamic gamma system with hyper-sensibility of the spindle receptors which are an expression of hyper-reflective tendinous reflexes.

The inter-neuronal system described by Renshaw constitutes the determining element of facilitation and inhibitory actions on the alpha motoneuron.

If one excepts myotatic, monosynaptic reflexes (reflex of Hoffmann) Renshaw's system controls and modulates all entering impulses before their arrival at the alpha motoneuron. It is also influenced by the activity of the alpha motoneurons themselves which receive recurrent collaterals. The other medullary inter-neurons form multiple circuits which are

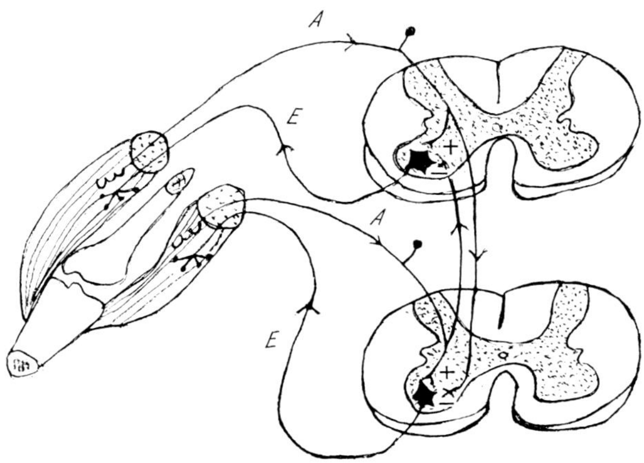

Fig. 2. Myotatic reflex and inhibiting reflex (after Morin). + Facilitation, — inhibition, *A* afferent sensory fiber, *E* motor efferent fiber

responsible for overall organization of the medullary reflexes and medullary integration.

2. Intersegmentary Control

Inter-segmentary control in normal man involves an inter-play of opposing groups not only for voluntary motor activity but also for the balance of tone. The law of reciprocal innervation (Sherrington[99]) explains the agonist-antagonist balance (Fig. 2).

Muscle contraction has as its origin hundreds of impulses which themselves act on the alpha motoneuron, assuring the tonic and phasic regulation of the muscle concerned. In addition these impulses will reach the adjacent medullary segments above and below where they have a suppressor effect on the myotatic reflex, causing the release of antagonist muscular groups.

This phenomenon is important; these spinal reflexes disappear in spinal man (Dimitrijevic and Nathan [21, 22]) with loss of reciprocal innervation to hyperactivity of motoneurons; thus all extero- or proprio-ceptive stimulation reinforces alpha hypertonus. This reinforcement is evident in the directly stimulated territory (reinforcement of spasticity by chronic exteroceptive or proprioceptive stimulation, such as bladder infections, pressure sores . . . etc.) but in incomplete medullary lesions there is diffusion above and below the stimulated zone, thus transmitting the hyperexcitability of all alpha motoneurons to a distance from the medullary sector stimulated.

In spastic man, posterior radiculotomy reduces facilitation impulses, resulting not only in hypotonia in the operated sectors, but also, a paradoxical reduction of spasticity in regions not affected by the radiculotomy (Gros and Ouaknine[42]).

The quantitative effect is proportional to the extent of the posterior radiculotomy and can be observed up to the bulbar region.

3. Supra-Segmental Control

Ablation of the cortex (Fulton[35]) or pyramidotomy in chimpanzees and other apes (Tower and Hines) results in flaccid paralysis of the limbs.

A deficit of cortico-extrapyramidal pathways renders hemiplegia spastic and results in a complete disorganization of motor activity. The influence of cortico-extrapyramidal fibers is greater in alpha motoneurons controlling the voluntary motor activity of intrinsic muscles of the hand and extensor digitorum communis.

This explains why a hemiplegic patient shows more severe affection of the extensors of the wrist and fingers and small muscles of the hand.

Absence of inhibitory functions of supra-spinal and cortical structures produces increased reflex activity of antigravity muscles (physiological extensors) particularly myotatic reflex activity, and is manifested in the form of strongly increased tone and involuntary movements such as clonus.

On the other hand, absence of facilitatory cortical functions related particularly to monosynaptic pathways, gives rise to cessation of inhibitory effects on antagonist muscles since the inability of muscles to contract interferes with the mechanism of reciprocal innervation.

Supra-medullary structures at the same time act on the gamma and alpha systems whose activities they control and inhibit.

The cortex controls above all, the dynamic system, the sub-cortical centres, the static mechanisms. The Paleo-Cerebellum exerts an inhibitory action on the cerebral cortex; its ablation results in hyperactivity of alpha motoneurons and spasticity which persists after posterior radiculotomy.

These neuro-physiological mechanisms have a biophysical basis which are better understood since the works of Eccles[24, 25, 26].

They help us to understand the action of pharmacological agents. Recurrent inhibition (Renshaw) is dependant on mediators (G. A. B. A. Glycocolle—Glycine).

Benzodiazepines would reinforced presynaptic inhibition.

Besides this segmental control, tonus regulation is dependant on central inhibiting influences, among them the Nigro-striatal, Dopaminergic system.

4. Laboratory Investigations

Neuro muscular laboratory investigation can be used as to complement clinical examination: Electro myogram, study of mono synaptic or poly synaptic reflexes.

In Figs. 4 and 5 are shown the results obtained in a normal subject and in a case of spasticity, by study of the cycle of excitability to double stimuli and by recording the recruitment curve.

From a practical point of view, although interesting, this cannot replace in value a minute clinical evaluation, whose results are plotted on the spastic study chart.

Since its origin (Foerster 1908) the Neuro-Surgery of the spastic has inspired animal experimentation and given rise to neuro-physiological hypothesis. In addition, conditions which give rise to spasticity, means of prevention, and ways of limiting their inconveniences are better understood. Lastly the number of pharmacological agents has increased. In listing the various medical and surgical treatments and their areas of overlap, one begins to understand the reason for the variety of principles followed and the therapeutic actions proposed.

III. The Natural History of Spasticity

Spasticity is present, to a variable degree, in a wide spectrum of neurological conditions:

Infantile hemiplegia, Infantile Palsy,

Cerebral or medullary lesions (traumatic, vascular, degenerative . . . etc.).

The common point is a lesion of the common motor pathway whatever its level, cortical, subcortical or medullary, and a lesion of extrapyramidal pathways.

On the other hand, spasticity will not appear in lesions affecting the alpha motoneuron, lesions of the posterior roots, of the long sensory tracts and cerebellar nuclei.

The association of lesions encountered in these two groups (notably in degenerative diseases) results in complex clinical pictures.

1. The Spastic Child

The younger the child, the more cerebral lesions disturb acquisition of normal motor patterns: sitting, grasping, standing, walking and talking.

Normal psychomotor patterns are acquired from imitation of environmental stimuli.

When the child attempts to move, there is obstruction due to improper tonic control. The child therefore slowly structures pathological motor patterns which use the existing tonic state to accomplish the desired motor function. These pathologic patterns will give similar clinical pictures whatever the etiology.

In the child, neonatal neurological damage and its consequences ought to be investigated during the first year of life, at which time therapeutic steps to prevent spasticity can be instigated; these will limit the development of abnormal motor patterns which manifest themselves in greater or lesser degree in the clinical picture of Little's disease. This supposes reeducation at the family level up to the age of 3 or 4, followed by admission to a specialized centre where reeducation can be pursued hand in hand with schooling.

Even under the best conditions spasticity will nevertheless disappear but under these conditions its consequences on the locomotor system are moderated.

On the other hand, left to his own devices the child will develope a variety of pathological conditions affecting motor adaptation, with early presentation of orthopaedic complications.

Where tonic disequilibrium is present only active rehabilitation methods are proposed (Bobath K, B 9) at present.

1.1. Investigations

Fundamental elements ought to be considered.

1.1.1. The I.Q. level and the psychological attitude vis-à-vis the illness. All therapy supposes an active participation, failing this, therapy will have to be limited in its aim as will be the therapeutic outcome.

1.1.2. Evaluation of functional adaptation: We recognize 4 degrees: total dependence, partial dependence, independence and active life.

Evaluation should specify: if walking is impossible, possible with a cane, with or without an apparatus.

This functional analysis synthesises the total capabilities of the child and upon it therapeutic suggestions and their possibilities will be based.

1.1.3. Analytical evaluation: Examination of balance retaining actions and straightening up is absolutely necessary if the future possibilities for walking are to be correctly estimated. This influences all decisions concerning surgical treatment.

Spasticity in the child is rarely symmetrical and on each side it will be noted that the lower limb is more severely affected than the upper, and there is usually imbalance between extensor and flexo-muscles, the pattern of Little's disease being generally observed.

At this stage it is fundamental that the analysis should consider spasticity from the point of view of its possible utility or handicap.

1.2. Useful or Handicapping Spasticity

Useful spasticity concerns those anti-gravity muscles which are necessary for standing up and walking: Gluteus medius, maximus and the quadriceps. They can be a major source of voluntary muscle power and alone will permit the patient to stand erect.

Handicapping spasticity occurs where a tonic disequilibrium is created between different groups of muscles. Two of its constituents may be:

a) hyperactive gamma tone which in general acts on certain muscle groups and not on their antagonists, resulting in the restriction of joint movement.

b) Gamma phasic hyperactivity which is characterized by excessive osteotendinous reflex activity, resulting in increased tension, of such a degree as to produce violent epileptiform jerking movements of the lower limbs.

The two components are often associated in the same patient.

In such a case evaluation of underlying voluntary motor activity is difficult. Masked function may become apparent after the reduction of the spasticity.

Posture of adductor flexion, internal rotation of the hip is a source of pain, of coxavalga then progressive luxation of the joint.

Hypertonus of the quadriceps femoris results in lengthening of the patellar ligament which reduces the efficacy of the muscle.

Hypertonus of the sural triceps and tibialis posterior results in dislocation of the joints of the foot, starting as a reducible equino varus, the opposing forces of the sural triceps and the components that maintain posture interact in such a way as to produce falling of the arch of the foot with subluxation of the talus and a painful, irreducible talus valgus foot (Fig. 3).

Handicapping spasticities can be summarized according to 4 dominant deleterious effects:

1. late onset of motor development,
2. inefficacy of antagonist muscles,
3. articular disequilibrium and their orthopaedic consequences,
4. evolution or non-evolution of the spasticity.

1.3. Codification of the Problems

Methods involving functional reeducation of the spastic child enable stabilization of the condition in a great number and facilitate social adaptation. The child usually reaches a level where he ceases to make progress, or where reeducation is no longer effective, or where the handicapping elements of the spasticity come to the foreground.

The use of a standardized examination code for spasticity permits chronological evaluation and objective grading of his state.

The same code ought to be used by centres of reeducation and Neuro-Surgical clinics interested in the problems of spasticity. Therapeutic decisions will be made directly from this chart.

2. The Adult Spastic

The many causes of spasticity in the adult cover numerous facts of neurology.

Diseases of motor function and spasticity are to be found associated with a wide variety of conditions with equally different sequelae such as cerebral hemiplegia, trauma, acute medullary lesions, and a number of degenerative diseases.

2.1. Period of Recovery

During the period of recovery of a hemiplegia, before the return of any voluntary muscular activity, actual muscle tone will appear in the diaphragm and the anti-gravity muscles of the lower limb, contrasting with the dominance of the flexors in the upper limb. The return of voluntary motor function when it occurs, diminishes the significance of this pathological pattern; if recovery is insufficient or non existent, hypertonus will increase, the patient will be able to bear weight on the lower limbs only because of the spasticity of these anti-gravitic muscles.

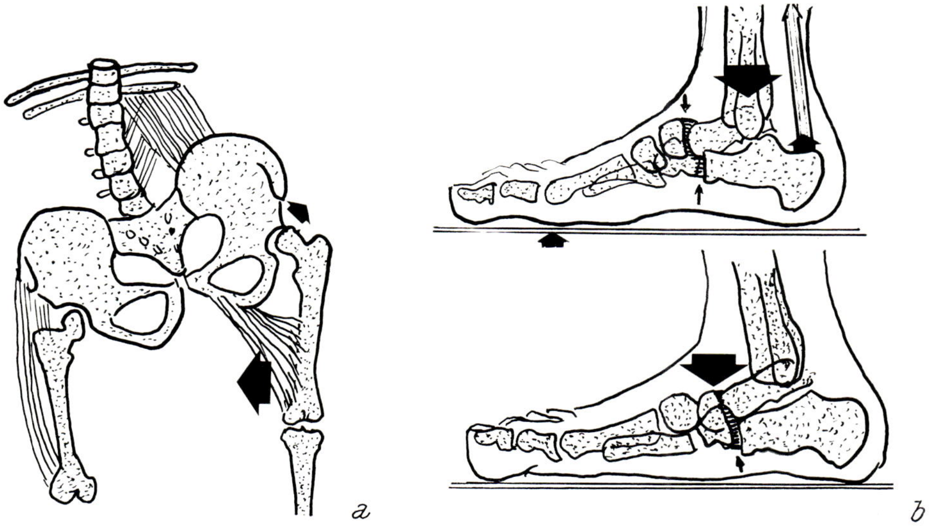

Fig. 3. Spasticity endangering joints. a) Adduction, . flexion type spasticity, = risk of hip dislocation. b) Surae muscle spasticity, = talus valgus, : tarso-metatarsyal dislocation

Concurrent elements which tend to increase the incapacity in spastic hemiplegia are as follows: the frequency of painful associated phenomena, an attitude of tonic flexion, fixation of the wrist and fingers, rendering the hand useless and unaesthetic, an incapacitating spasticity of the foot in equino-varus with complete loss of effective antagonist function.

Spasticity resulting from traumatic lesions of the spine, as in chronic diseases of the spine, results in different clinical syndromes according to the level and type of lesion.

One must distinguish the different types, for as we shall see later, they justify different surgical procedures.

Segmentary medullary lesions can produce spasticity when situated at the level of the cervical or thoracic spine, isolating the caudal part of the spinal cord.

The lower the lesion, the less likely is this condition to be found. It must be remembered that the higher is the lesion on the cord the larger will be the distal area of the cord submitted to tonic afferent impulses. Also there is direct relationship between the extent of the lesion and the degree of spasticity produced by reason of loss of the inhibitory influences of the common pyramidal pathway.

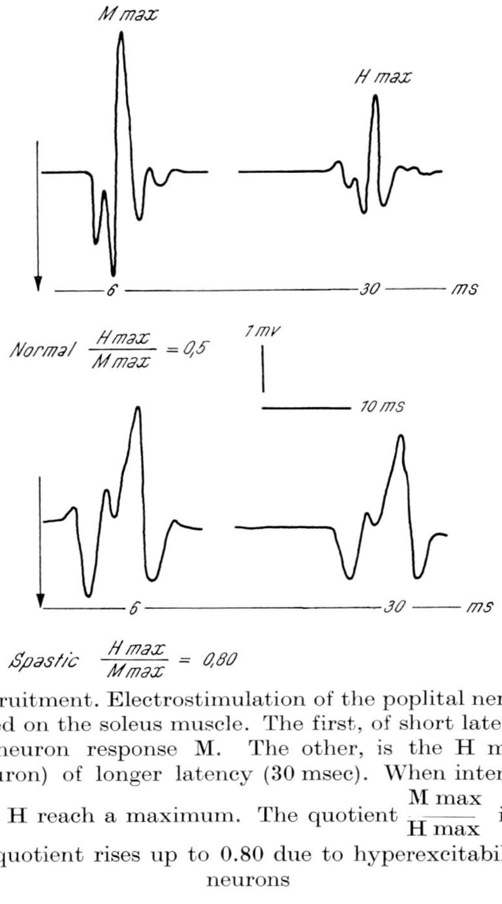

Fig. 4. Curve of recruitment. Electrostimulation of the poplital nerve, gives two types of responses recorded on the soleus muscle. The first, of short latency (6 m sec) is the direct alpha motoneuron response M. The other, is the H monosynaptic reflex (1 a alpha motoneuron) of longer latency (30 msec). When intensity of stimulation is increased, M and H reach a maximum. The quotient $\frac{\text{M max}}{\text{H max}}$ is normally 0.5. In spastic cases this quotient rises up to 0.80 due to hyperexcitability of alpha motoneurons

With J. Benezech[6,11], we examined the initial stages of recovery by studying the cortical somatosensory evoked responses (C.E.P.), and the monosynaptic H reflex.

Initially in spinal shock, the H reflex disappears and it is not possible to evoke a cortical potential by peripheral stimulation.

Return of the H reflex is the first sign of spinal functional recovery below the lesion at a stage when the tendon reflexes are still absent and somatic potentials cannot be obtained.

24 hours later the presence of C.E.P. potentials announces the return of long tract functions, and by studying the recruitment curve H max/M max (normal: 0.5) and the H reflex in double stimulation a quantitative evalua-

tion of the return of tone and its accentuation right up to the stage of clinical hypertonus is possible (Fig. 4).

During the stage of hypertonus, hypoexcitability is noted the second H response being retarded, and needing an interval of 150 m before reaching the first in amplitude.

The passive progression towards spasticity shortens the delay of the response in double shock states which becomes less than 1000 milliseconds and is associated with an increased H max/M max ratio (Fig. 5).

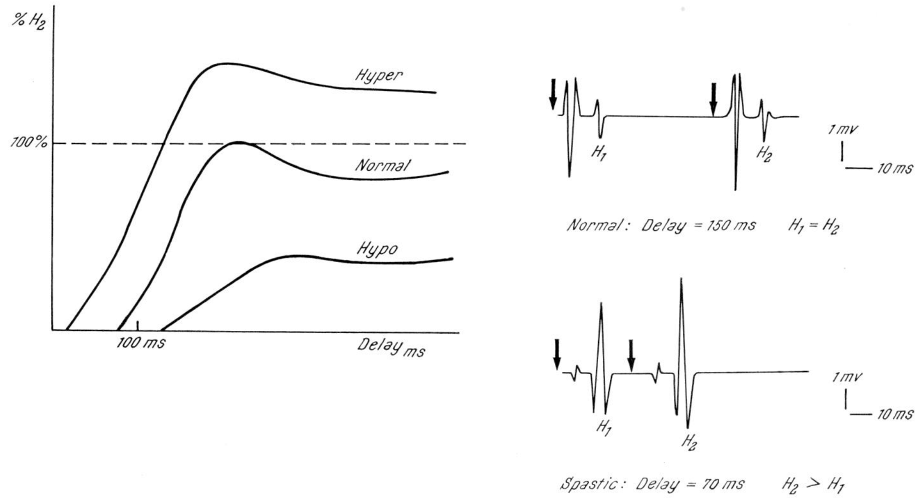

Fig. 5. Cycle of excitability (double stimulus). On normal subject, 2 electrics shocks applied on the poplital nerve need to be separated by a delay of 100 to 150 msec, to give the identical H reflex. In cases of spasticity, this delay is shorter than 100 m/sec and the second H reflex reachs a higher amplitude than the first

We shall now consider the different types of spastic paraplegia most frequently seen.

2.2. Spasticity in "Extension"

Spasticity in extension is usually seen in lesions situated at the level of the cervical or dorsal spine; we should consider it a usually avoidable complication in a patient who has been correctly treated from the moment of his accident, to a stage of stabilization which can vary between 2 to 12 months, depending on the case.

On the other hand it is almost invariably seen in circumstances where significant noxious stimulation has been allowed to develop: bed sores, bladder infection, pressure sores, articular immobility.

Dominance of the anti-gravity muscles over the flexor muscles causes fixed hypertonus at the hip, the knee in extension, and the foot in the equinovarus deformity. Frequently hypertonus of the flexors and adductors of the hip results in a variation of this position with crossing of the legs.

The intensity of the spasticity renders the sitting position uncomfortable, and nursing hygiene difficult, frequently there are, in addition, painful cramps and disturbing jerking movements.

Spasticity of the bladder causes a reduction in its capacity with frequent and incomplete micturition ureteral reflux with upper urinary tract sequelae.

Evolution of the spasticity will thereafter vary. In the absence of cutaneous or bladder complications and other intercurrent illnesses, post-traumatic tonic equilibrium should stabilize in the year following the accident, but if at any time there is significant stimulation from noxious impulses this equilibrium can be disturbed.

Spasticity symptomatic of cervicoarthrosic myelopathies are often intense in contrast with the discreteness of the neurological signs and deficiencies produced.

Prior to the development of major motor deficits, spasticity in extension is for a long period the dominant complaint in the progressive spinal paralysis of Strümpell-Lorrain.

The spasticity of disseminated sclerosis is very variable and is not typical at the onset of the disease. Its course over the years is characterized particularly by the accompaniment of painful paroxysms; frequently there is an evolution towards the appearance of dominant cutaneo-reflex activity with a tendency to triple withdrawal, followed by paraplegia in flexion.

2.3. *Spasticity in "Flexion"*

If one admits that spasticity is the reflection of a pathological exaggeration of the stretch reflex, it is then necessary to understand why a paraplegia in flexion can develop.

It must be recalled that the interneurone system of Renshaw is subject to an influx of many stimuli usually resulting in increased alpha activity. The conditions which give rise to spasticity in flexion are observed in cases of strong nociceptive influences either from skin, bladder or joints, poorly tolerated apparatus or in medullary lesions affecting the interneurone system.

"This type of hypertonus is not abolished by posterior rhizotomy and is not due to an exaggerated myotatic reflex" (I. M. Tarlov[115]). It is due to impulse discharge of motor neurones, which, deprived of interneural influences, become spontaneously active" (I. M. Tarlov).

Paraplegia in flexion produces incapacitating consequences: lying in bed is difficult, sitting is impossible, there are frequent paroxysms in flexion, a serious risk of pressure sores, of painful phenomena and progressive articular dislocation.

3. *Spasticity and Involuntary Movements*

Spasticity is frequently associated with abnormal movements (dystonia, dyskinesia, athetosis), when the lesion is situated in the brain stem and the sub-cortical nuclei. This situation is frequently encountered in infantile palsy associated with neonatal anoxia and kernicterus.

It is found also in the long term sequelae of cranial trauma associated with prolonged coma and reflects primary or secondary meso-diencephalic lesions.

The superimposition of these problems on spasticity makes the evaluation of the latter difficult, having not only a different anatomical target but also a different etiology, and being influenced by various affective factors. The two problems also respond to quite different therapeutic measures.

In such cases, dyskinetic or dystonic symptomatology associated with spasticity, would require specific treatment.

IV. Neurosurgery of Spasticity

There is no miracle operation for the cure of spasticity. Operations which are suggested were all inspired either by experimental work done on animals or by pathophysiological hypotheses.

For didactic reasons the different types of operations will be described without strict respect to chronology.

We shall deal successively with neurotomies, rhizotomies, cordotomies and more central interventions (brain and cerebellum).

1. Neurotomies

These were among the earliest operations to be performed: Stoffel 1912[110] in the treatment of deformities of the foot in cerebral palsy. Since then, the action on peripheral nerves has been produced either by Procaine infiltration in muscle (Walshe[124]) or in motor end-plates (Matthews and Rushworth[69]) or by infiltration of alcohol into motor areas (Tardieu[112]). Neurotomies in the true sense were used by Silfverskiold[106] and classified by Phelps[85].

In fact the aim is different in the two cases. Novocaine infiltrations have a short lived effect whereas alcohol injections have a longer lasting effect on alpha fibers, when 96% alcohol is used (Tardieu[114]); spasticity can disappear for a period of 1 to 6 months after injection into the motor areas of the sural muscles without a notable reduction in motor activity.

We have reapplied the technique of neurotomy because we consider that the results obtained can be improved if the general principles of treatment of spasticity are scrupulously respected, if operative stimulation under micro-dissection is used and if the extent of neurotomy is sufficient.

The investigation of spasticity, as we outlined above, will allow for a more precise decision about the application of neuro-surgical intervention in relationship to the development of the disease or the failure of medical and physiotherapeutic measures.

It also allows for a precise descriptive analysis of muscles affected by handicapping spasticity and the development of eventual contractures.

The therapeutic application can now be considered.

Treatment of the spastic equinovarus foot:

This is the most common case and it is easy to note which muscles are affected: the gastrocnemius, the soleus, the posterior tibialis, and the common flexors of the toes.

Exposure of the sciatic nerve in the internal popliteal region, microdissection of its branches and operative stimulation will enable the charting of the different muscular branches on their way to the muscles and also those which come together to form the posterior tibial nerve (Fig. 6).

Indications for neurotomy in the upper limb are rare but we have obtained an improvement in flexion of the elbow by a neurotomy of the triceps, which allowed the patient to feed himself (spastic tetraparesis).

Experience shows that branches innervating the spastic muscles are excitable at a lower threshold than that of the non spastic muscles, so that each branch ought to be resected to 4/5ths or 5/6ths of its volume if a permanent result is to be achieved, but the conservation of 1/5th or 1/6th of the fibers is enough to save voluntary motor activity.

Our experience is concerned with 46 patients followed over 5 years. They include tonic gamma spasticity, in hemiplegics, paraplegics or in IMC. Infantile palsy.

Immediate Effect

Study of spasticity shows that foremost:

1. The stretch reflex is lost or considerably reduced in the operated sectors, as could be predicated.

2. Hypertonus of the non operated antagonist muscles is likewise reduced: extensor muscles of the knee, dorsi-flexors of the foot. Recovery of use and power in the quadriceps is always noted by the patients. In every case the reciprocal innervation law of Sherrington has been verified, decrease of the spasticity in the agonists liberates motor function in the antagonists.

Late Effect

There is regression of the painful phenomena which are frequently associated with spasticity. Reequilibrium of the foot and of the toes at rest becomes evident when walking, in particular for the spastic hemiplegic, who is able to walk without faltering. Increased osteo-tendinous reflexes in the operated zone clear.

The patient becomes aware of his new motor function and with the help of analytical rehabilitation continues to make progress whereas before the operation he remained stabilized without hope of progress.

Electro-physiological exploration (study of the H max/M max ratio, integrated electromyography will confirm these results.

In fact physiologically, neurotomies are complex operations for they cut, in variable quantities according to the nerves:

1. the motor fibers;

2. the sensory fibers I a, I b, II and III (Loyd's classification) acting at the same time on the afferent and efferent pathways of myotatic reflex.

Later we shall discuss the place of this benign surgery in the therapeutic armamentarium of spasticity.

2. *Radiculotomy*

It is encouraging to think of the experience gained by Foerster[28] in 1908, when publishing 62 cases of posterior radiculotomies in the treatment of spasticity, using in man the surgical procedures performed by Sherrington in the cat.

The freedom of movement obtained in the legs allowed children to walk who previously were too spastic to do so.

The long term results published in 1913 confirmed the earlier report, despite a slight return of spasticity.

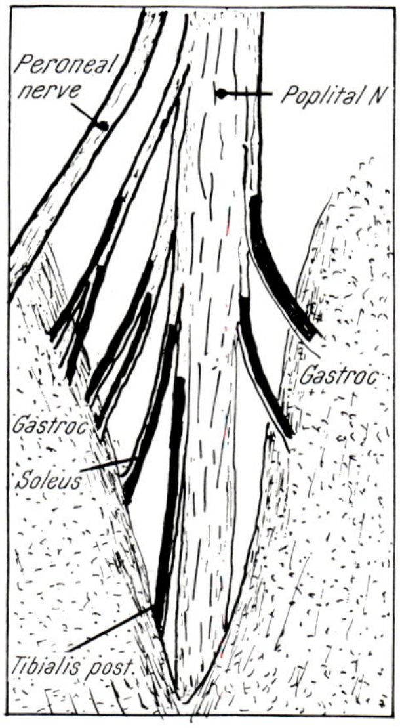

Fig. 6. Poplital sectorial neurotomy. Neurotomy 4/5 of the motor rami of the spastic muscles according to the clinical testing of spasticity and to the result of electrostimulation during operation spasticity involving gastrochemius, soleus, and tibialis posterior muscles

Despite the disappearance or reduction of spasticity, the method has been criticized on the grounds of producing sensory disorders, in particular a loss of proprioreceptive sensation, transforming the spastics into "tabetics".

It is also criticized for suppressing all the muscle tone in the lower limbs, which some patients had learnt to use to overcome their incapacity.

The complexity of the problems posed is such that it is not possible to accept or to refute all these criticisms: nevertheless there were failures or functional aggravations and even though these were exceptional, they were sufficient to discredit the method.

Many modifications have been applied to the original techniques of Foerster.

In 1967, then in 1972, we published the results obtained by posterior selective radicotomies in 62 cases; with a follow up of over 18 years.

The P.S.R. operation covers the root levels L 1–S 1, after laminectomy of L 1 and L 2. There are between 20 and 30 posterior rootlets representing L 1, L 2, L 3, L 4, L 5 and S 1. The resection is carried out on 4 posterior rootlets out of 5, the 1/5th of rootlets preserved allows one at the same time to respect the radicular arteries and the peripheral sensation.

2.1. Direct Effect

The effect on spasticity was immediate, rapid muscle stretching no longer producing spastic contractions, muscular equilibrium appearing at rest—decreasing the risk of progressive luxation.

Crisis of contractures, or painful spasms ceased or diminished in intensity. However, the result was incomplete if associated musculo-tendinous contractions existed.

Conservation of sensation in the lower limbs was the most remarkable fact: careful examination showed some areas of relative hypoesthesia in 22 patients out of 62.

40 patients did not have any abnormality of sensation on examination.

Abnormalities of sphincter function were only observed if the radiculotomy did not respect the S 2 and S 3 rootlets.

2.2. "Distant" Effect

The distant effect of PSR has been studied in 25 cases of infantile palsy: 18 spontaneously noticed an improvement of the upper limbs and of speech. In 14 patients presenting various degrees of hypertonus of the upper limbs, 9 noticed greater flexibility of the hand; writing and self feeding were easier.

An improvement in speech was noted in 5 cases in relation to phonation and articulation.

Theses facts must be compared to those published by R. Heimburger[52] who obtained excellent reduction of spasticity of the lower limbs, after posterior radiculotomies performed on the three first cervical roots.

It appears that reduction of afferent sensory impulses, whatever its level, has two complementary effects, a direct and sharp reduction of the gamma tonic stimuli at the segmental level, and a diffuse, more limited decrease of spasticity, away from the level of radiculotomy. This "distant" effect appears to be related to the quantitative reduction of all stimulation transmitted by the medullary interneurones.

Late results ought not to be evaluated until the patient has been reeducated for 6 to 12 months in a specialized centre. Overall improvement was noted in 75% of the patients operated.

Rehabilitation helps the patient to acquire new motor patterns which will replace the pathological ones suppressed by the operation.

If the patient is unable to collaborate with his reeducation (mental retardation, depression etc.) he will only passively benefit from his operation and will make no functional progress. This underlines the necessity for a complete evaluation of the situation before making a definite decision.

Good results are seen in infantile cerebral spasticity and in spastic paraplegics. These improvements continue to progress during one year. Relapse is apparent if rehabilitation is stopped, if the patient develops urinary infection, decubitus pressure sores or articular complications.

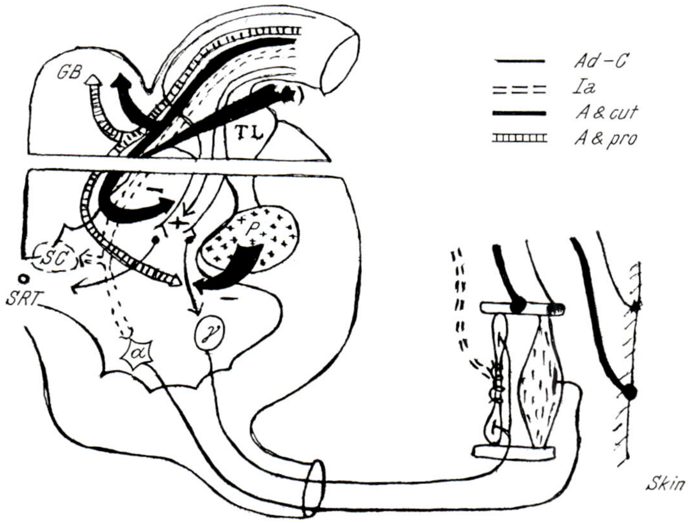

Fig. 7. Systematization of fibers at the level of the radiculo-medullar junction (after Sindou). *GB* Goll and Burdach, *SC* origin of the spino cerebellar tract, *TL* Lissauer tract, *P* pyramidal tract, *SRT* spino-reticulo-thalamic tract, *Ad–C* small size fibers, on the surface of the root, *Ia* large size fibers, in central position, * posterior selective radicellotomy

Less favourable results are seen in degenerative diseases with spasticity, either because of the diffuse character of the medullary lesions or their evolution.

2.3. Failure or Deterioration

The 25% failure rate is normally due to errors in case selection, particularly with over evaluation of voluntary motor power.

One case of functional worsening particularly impressed us:

A male, 40 years old, spastic paraplegia in extension of medical origin. Complications: 1. sitting position difficult, 2. walking possible with two crutches, the support being borne on the two great toes giving a swinging walk.

Selective posterior radiculotomy 4/5th bilateral of L 1 to S 1 was performed. Despite a year's reeducation, muscular function remained very poor. Walking was only possible with two Phelps braces. Analytically the spasticity was diminished; functionally the situation was worse. Such a failure demonstrates clearly that spasticity in itself cannot be considered as a condition automatically justifying its reduction, but as a complex picture of which a part can be used functionally by the patient although a part remains harmful.

These reasons have led us to review and modify the technique we initially used.

3. Posterior Radiculotomy: New Techniques

Three modifications of posterior radiculotomy have been proposed aiming to conserve its efficacy without the risk of reducing functionally useful aptitudes.

3.1. Posterior "Rhizidiotomy" of Sindou et al.

Sindou *et al.*[107, 108] proposed limiting the section made in the posterior rootlets, to the fiber A delta and C and the fibers I a, saving the A beta fibers, going to the lemniscus and which have an inhibitory effect (Fig. 7).

A delta, C and I a fibers have a facilitatory effect on gamma motoneurons, and are laterally situated. A beta fibers are more postero-medially placed.

Thus, a correctly situated section, at a depth of 1 to 2 mm, at the level of entry of each rootlet, should theoretically allow a selective effect on spasticity, saving part of the deep sensory pathways.

Under the microscope, isolation of each rootlet is easy at the cervical level, but very dificult in the lumbar region where the posterior rootlets are grouped without discontinuity.

Sindou operated on 12 patients complaining of severe SP, whose nursing had become difficult from to the grossly abnormal position of their limbs. He obtained in 7 cases of paraplegia of "flexion" type, 5 early good results and 2 failures; results were good in 2 out of 3 cases of painful spasticity of the upper limb.

Such cases appear to be the best indication for this technique, since anatomical conditions are favorable at the cervical level.

3.2. Partial Posterior Rootlet Section of Guidetti and Fraioli

With the experience of the Foerster radiculotomy, Guidetti and Fraioli proposed to effect partial section of each posterior rootlet of the spastic limbs, in their posterior 2/3, close to the lateral posterior sulcus. The aim was to avoid the risk of any sensory deficit.

They operated on 26 patients, suffering from SP of perinatal etiology. Prior to the operation, all were able to walk, 2 were independent; all had good intellectual level.

The best results (11 out of 15) were observed in the cases whose SP was increased by involuntary movements. Improvement was poor, when voluntary movements increased SP (9); recurrence appeared in one case; hyperactive stretch reflexes cleared partially or totally.

Reduction of deep sensibility was observed in only one case. Distant, supralesional effect was evident on the upper limbs, speach was improved 3 times and mastication once.

This conservation of sensory function led Guidetti and Fraioli to think that posterior section saves the ventral part of the posterior rootlets where the proprioceptive sensory fibers must be situated.

3.3. Sectorial Posterior Radiculotomy (Gros[41])

We have tried to observe 3 principles:
Effective reduction of SP.
Protection of the tone of muscles necessary for walking or sitting.
Conservation of proprioceptive sensibility.

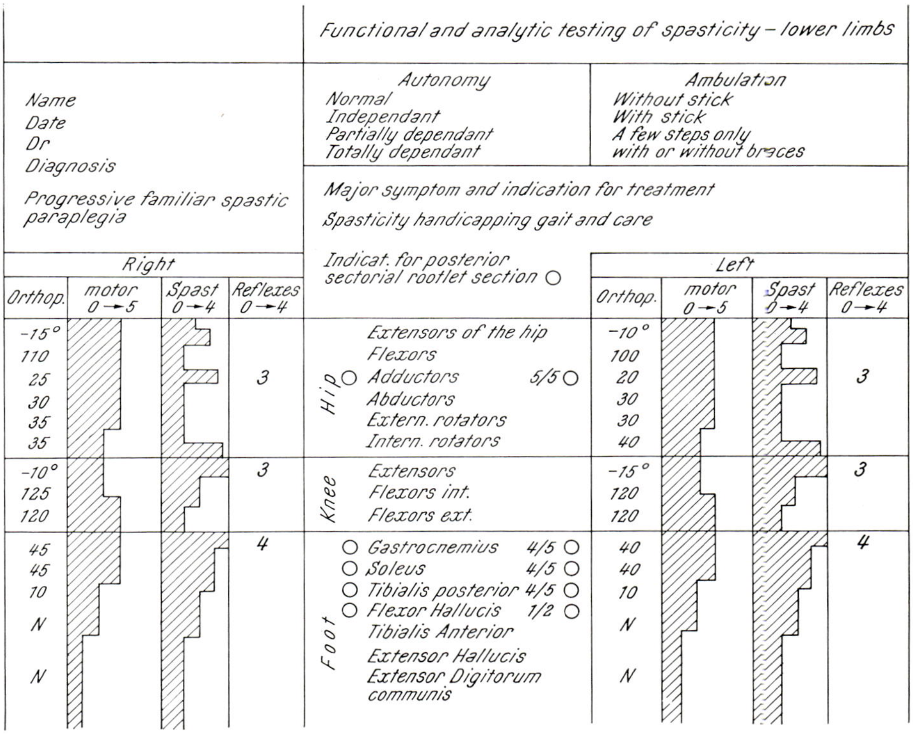

Fig. 8. Functional and analytic testing of spasticity—lower limbs

This pre-supposes a new approach in diagnosis and requires a fresh technology.

Clinical evaluation of each case is made by an interdisciplinary team where the physical therapists and the neurosurgeons work regularly together.

All the factors to be checked, must be summarized in a special chart, using a pre-established code, enabling the evolution of the disease to be catalogued (Fig. 8).

3.3.1. Factorial Checking

The following points must be studied:
social adaptation (4 grades)
mental attitude
I Q

orthopaedic study: muscular retractions, joint state
motor voluntary control (5 grades)
spasticity
  topography and intensity (4 grades)
  useful or handicapping muscles

Evaluation of involuntary motor power is difficult in patients with high grade of SP. We evaluate this hidden potential involuntary power, when any doubt exists, by checking the patient at the initial stage of lumbar subarachnoidal spinal anesthesia:

8 cg of Procaïne are used, the patient lying on his back immediately after injection. The initial action of Procaïne on posterior roots and spindles is to suppress the spasticity and for 3 to 10 minutes it does not affect the motor roots. This latency allows the Physical Therapist to check voluntary motor power.

The spasticity chart underlines all the factors necessary for treatment and if surgery is justified, it contains all the elements for the "surgical programme".

3.3.2. Operative Technique

The patient under general endotracheal anaesthesia, is placed on his left side, allowing two teams to work together, the Physical Therapist being placed in front with access to the lower limbs and perineum.

The approach is made from the right side, the spinous processes being cut at their base and separated with the muscular masses of the left side; the articular facettes are strictly protected, the level of laminectomy corresponds to D 12–L 1 and eventually to L 2 if the conus is in a low position.

Functional charting of the posterior rootlets:

The posterior roots exposed comprise about 20 to 25 rootlets, which must be isolated and stimulated to obtain a good map of their function, as no precise anatomical reference is obtainable, due to the limited surgical approach (Fig. 9).

Stimulation is monopolar, by rectangular waves at low frequency 40 to 50 Hz, 0.8 to 3 volts, 1 millisecond.

Results of stimulation are analysed by the neurophysiologist, either directly or with electromyography. Contraction of the anal sphincter is noted; occasional bladder contractions are observed with cystomanometry.

This evaluation extending from the abdominal to the sural muscles builds a map of the rootlets; those having a specific function are marked by coloured threads. Identification may be difficult; the responses are more short lasting and obtained at a lower threshold for spastic sectors than for the others.

Separation between the adductor rootlets and those of the quadriceps femoris is sometimes impossible by stimulation of posterior rootlets; one must therefore look for the motor root of the adductor, mark its exit, and then start from this level down.

There are often asymmetries between the level of the two sides. Normally there are 2 to 3 rootlets for the adductors, 4 to 6 for the quadriceps, 5 to 6 for the calf muscles, whilst the foot and toe flexors appear to have only 1 to 2.

Posterior rootlet section is decided in relation to the pre-established program and to the mapping of the posterior rootlets.

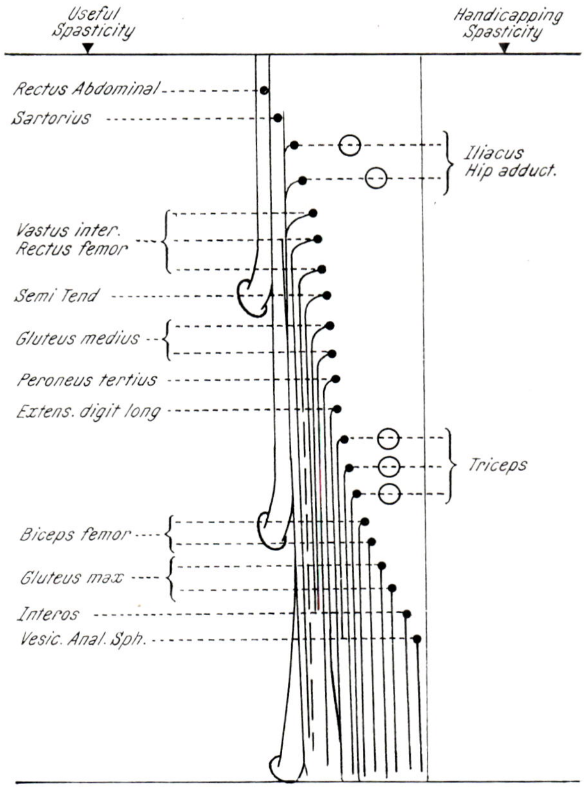

Fig. 9. Drawing of posterior rootlet stimulations. ◯ Sectorial posterior rootlet section

For regions considered as handicapping, rootlet sections are made saving only 1/5th or less of their fibers.

Sectors of useful spasticity situated above or below this area are entirely preserved.

It is therefore a sectorial radiculotomy which is done "on request" and conserves the reflex arcs of the gluteus-maximus quadriceps, etc. . . .

The operation does not modify bladder function as it stops at S 1.

We do not place a urinary catheter during the post-operative period and the patient gets up on the 4th day.

3.3.3. Results

Favorable results were obtained in 22 cases of SPR operated cases. Gamma tonic and phasic hyperactivity were immediately reduced in the treated sector; moreover the result on the antagonist muscles was evident since it was then possible to estimate precisely voluntary motor activity.

A supra-segmentary effect is only noted when the number of sectioned rootlets is large.

The quality related rapidity of post-operative recuperation, is to the topography and the number of sectors treated. For limited spasticity, the rootlet section is limited and recuperation is rapid; for child spastic from cerebral palsy rootlet section must cover several sectors, new motor patterns develop slowly and need several months of reeducation before the child benefits completely from the new motor possibilities revealed by the tonic reequilibrium.

A certain grade of hypertonus returns and osteo-tendinous reflexes can be observed if the operation has been too limited, either deliberately or because of error in the electrophysiological marking.

The functional results are satisfactory, often permitting walking without appliances; defective postures are remarkably corrected by the tonic reequilibrium, as long as the orthopaedic lesions are reversible.

Pain usually ceases at the same time as spasticity.

We have performed 9 fractional posterior radiculotomies for upper limb spasticity.

The anatomical disposition of the cervical roots aids their stimulation and in the preparation of a pre-operative map. For hemiplegics the operation is unilateral; in the majority of cases the aim is to obtain reduction of spasticity in flexion for the wrist and fingers, for this spasticity is often painful and accompanied by important sensury deficits.

Successive stimulation of rootlets from C 6 to T 1 allow the determination of which control extension of the wrist and fingers and which control flexion.

This allows one to map rootlets' function and to perform partial section of those, controlling handicapping hyperflexion.

For a spastic elbow, which usually limits the movements necessary to reach the mouth, rootlets subversing extension of the elbow must be sought and partially cut.

The results, however limited they may be, are very promising; pain ceases and the resumption of reeducation permits a progressive tonic reequilibrium.

These results may be compared to those obtained by Heimburger; this author performed C 2–C 3 bilateral posterior radiculotomies and observed a partial but diffuse reduction of spasticity.

4. Anterior Radiculotomy

Pollock and Davis experiments on spasticity obtained by vertebral and carotid ligation in the cat showed that it was not modified by posterior radiculotomy, but that it yielded to anterior radiculotomy; showing that in this case SP is due to alpha hyperactivity alone, the alpha neurones having lost all inhibitory control.

Anterior radiculotomy was recommended by Monro in 1945 where it could be proved that the extent of medullary destruction excluded all possibility of preserved motor power.

Thus I. M. Tarlov[115] suppressed a persistent severe hypertonus after the failure of posterior radiculotomy; the low spinal cord showed diffuse lesion. He writes: "The most important aspect of this is a clear cut proof that damage to spinal interneurones may cause severe hypertonus in man, . . . that is unaffected by posterior root section or spinal cord transsection."

We have described these anatomical conditions in chapter III. We have had to treat 5 cases at this dramatic stage; recovery after anterior radiculoromy was simple, all hypertonus was suppressed and pressure sores healed rapidly.

5. *Myelotomy*

Scarff and Pool, Feld and Pecker performed posterior column resection with the aim of supression of the propioceptive afferent impulses from spastic sectors (1951).

Bischof[7,8] in 1951 performed a coronal section of the spinal cord in the ependymal plane T 11 to S 2. The section passed between the pyramidal tract behind and the spino-thalamic tract in front (Fig. 10).

Thus the sensory-motor reflex arc and the longitudinal system of the interneurones of Kölliker on which the polysynaptic reflex depends, were cut.

This operation was performed either by a unilateral or bilateral approach.

Out of 20 case histories published in 1962 by Tönnis and Bischof, the SP was regularly reduced but later reappeared in 5 cases. "Of the 20 patients 18 had been confined to be before the operation; only three remained bed patients after the operation and four were able to walk."

The evaluation of these spastic patients in aspect of motor potential was difficult; some of them seemed to have revealed involuntary movements unsuspected before the operation.

Bladder disorders were observed in some partial sections rather than in the large sections; some patients showing bladder hypertonus were improved.

P. D. Moyes[78] in 1969, published a study of 21 cases operated using Bischof's technique. It concerned patients with severe spasms in flexion; for 19 the results were good, 2 simply showed an improvement. Some patients observed difficulty in voluntary control of micturition. Some authors considered that the risk of injury to large pathways ought not to be underestimated and that the operation ought to be reserved for patients with complete transections of the spinal cord.

M. H. Pourpre[89] 1959, suggested performing the myelotomy after a posterior commissural myelotomy as deep as the ependyma (Fig. 10a).

This myelotomy in the form of a cross claims to respect the pyramidal fiber terminations and to section the sensory-motor reflex arc but at the same time cutting the spino-thalamic inflow generating spasticity.

The results obtained in 5 cases by Pourpre were comparable to those of Bischof (Fig. 10b).

Laitinen 1966[62], after having used Bischof's technique performed a section by introducing a myelotome in the sagittal plane which allowed a stylet to emerge at the desired point. The operation ought to be performed not less than 6 centimetres from the top of the cord and should

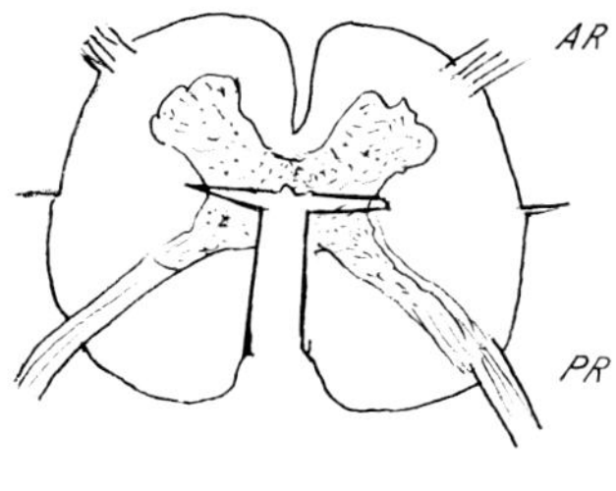

Fig. 10 a. Frontal myelotomy through posterior approach (Pourpre-Laitinen) *AR* anterior root, *PR* posterior root

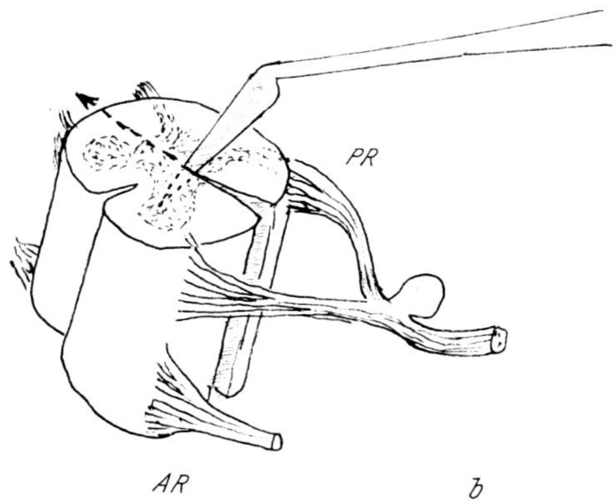

Fig. 10 b. Longitudinal myelotomy from T 12 to S 1 (Bischof)

respect the lowest 2 centimetres. In 5 cases, the initial results were satisfactory, SP reappeared 3 times. There were no bladder disorders of long duration.

A. Benedetti and C. Carbonin[4], using Laitinen's technique operated on 12 paraplegics (4 post-traumatic and 8 multiple sclerosis), each showing serious spasticity with contraction in flexion.

The operation improved, above all, the bedridden patients having defective posture of the lower limbs. There were three relapses. Three patients showed transitory incontinence before their bladder automatism returned.

In all the work published on myelotomy in the treatment SP, one must note the following essential features:

It is a difficult operation and may damage the large pathways subserving motor activity.

It has a lasting suppressive or reducing effect on SPr notably the painful SPr in flexion.

In some cases it may bring about lasting disturbances of micturition and erection.

All authors who have had the experience, state that it should be reserved for cases where the medullary lesions are complete or nearly so, and where the bladder function is compromised.

6. Central Operations

The spectacular strides of stereotatic surgery from 1960 onwards in the treatment of Parkinson's disease have proved that selective operations on the ventral and postero-ventral nuclei of the thalamus have an immediate and lasting action on tremor and rigidity. The operation had no effect on spasticity and other methods have been studied.

6.1. Dentatectomy—Dentatolysis

Delmas-Marsalet and van Bogaert (1935) showed that a dentate nucleus lesion can reduce rigidity and spasticity. Heimburger (1963), and subsequently numerous authors (Nashold[80], Krayenbühl and Siegfried 1969[61], Fraioli 1973[30], Verdie 1975[119]) performed stereotatic Dentatolysis. But it was not convincing and dentatectomy has gradually lost its adherents.

The role of the dentate nucleus in SP pathophysiology has not been proved with certainty. Studies of evoked cortical potentials from stimulation of the dentate nucleus have shown them to be recorded in the fronto-central regions (area 4 and 6) and in the parietal regions. It is considered that the dentate nucleus can influence muscular tonus via the dento-rubro-thalamo-cortical fibres (Jansen 1954) but a direct effect on the spinal projection pathway cannot be excluded. Fraioli and Guidetti[32] (88 cases) and J. Siegfried[104] (120 cases) studied the results of dentatectomy with great care. The authors admit favourable results in 1. 44% of Little's syndrome or infantile spastic hemiplegia, 2. 28% in uni or bilateral athetosis. Siegfried concludes his experience: "Stereotatic dentatectomy, in our hands, has never suppressed completely and lastingly the spasticity, but remains useful in certain cases."

Fraioli considers that dentatectomy must be bilateral to be efficient, but it cannot modify major spasticity, and it is ineffective if marked cortical atrophy exists. He concludes: "These syndromes which generally show a severe spasticity, will benefit more consistently from partial posterior spinal root and rootlet section".

6.2. Pulvinarolysis

The physiological role of the Pulvinar is not clearly known; it is a receptor for the parietal, occipital, temporal and cerebellar afferents.

Pulvinarolysis was initially suggested as a treatment for intractable pain (Cooper 1971), but on 36 cases operated on by the author he noted 19 satisfactory results for dystonia musculorum deformans, but only 7 "slight results" in 10 cases of infantile spastic hemiplegia.

Fraioli operated on 12 cases for mixed dyskinetic spastic syndromes. There were 3 failures, 7 improvements, 3 only moderate; phasic SP was improved but not tonic SP.

Siegfried noted that in 40 pulvinarolysis for treatment of pain, there was no reduction of pre-operative tonus. In 2 cases of pulvinarolysis for SP the result was not convincing.

Kanaka and Balasubramanian[59] operated on 7 cases of infantile spastic hemiplegia and considered the operation to be more effective than dentatectomy.

It appears that pulvinarolysis should not be considered as a reasonable treatment for spasticity except cases where pain could justify the operation.

V. Utilization of Electrical Functional Stimulations (EFS)

All preceding operations have tried to reduce the facilitatory influences acting on motor neurone activity by selective interruption of various pathways, or by influencing the motor-neurone activity itself, when the preceding operations have failed.

Animal experimentation and the results obtained in man, apart from the segmentary effect on the agonist and the antagonist muscles, have shown an important distant effect on other segments. It appears evident that these operations, even those seemingly very peripheral or localized, modify the entire spinal reflex activity.

A priori one could foresee that electrical stimulation (EFS) of the peripheral nervous system, apart from the immediate effect on the muscular region concerned, could have an effect on the antagonist musculature; experience has confirmed this.

Less foreseen was that a long term effect was likely to be observed in the form of a true reorganization of spinal function.

Liberson *et al.* (1961) had reported functional stimulation of skeletal muscles (peroneal nerve) in a hemiplegic patient[64, 65]. Stimulation was applied during the gait at the swing phase.

Peripheral nerve stimulation in animals had been extensively studied: McNeal (1973)[73], Pette, D., *et al.* (1973)[84], Al Amoods, W. S., *et al.* (1973), Riley, D. A. (1973)[94], Guth, L., *et al.* (1972)[49], Steinberger, W. W., *et al.* (1968)[109].

Human application of implanted electrodes was made by Jeglic, A., *et al.* (1967)[58], by McNeal (1973).

Gracanin, F., *et al.* published in 1972[40] their experience on EFS with skin surface electrodes applied mainly on the peroneal nerve (103 cases) and less frequently on radial or median nerves.

1. Technical Conditions

The generators employed use frequencies of 30 to 50 Hz.

The stimulus is rectangular; with pulse width from 0,3 to 1 ms, voltage from 4 to 50 volts and duration of stimulation from 500 to 2000 msec.

The output current can be adjusted and so adapted to each particular case.

1.1. Applications by Surface Bipolar Electrodes

By its superficial location at the neck of the fibula, the external popliteal nerve is easily accessible; as is the radial on the back of the forearm and the median at the wrist. The posterior tibial nerve and the trunk of the sciatic nerve are practically inaccessible.

Electrodes have a diameter of 1 to 2 cm^2. They are placed on the skin at intervals of 5 to 8 cm. The side of the electrode placed on the skin is covered with a special conducting paste to obtain good contact.

They are fixed with an easily removable bracelet or knee cap. The cutaneous tolerance varies according to the patients and the strength of the current. If there is burning sensation or intense tingling, the current must be decreased and it is then essential to achieve better contact with the nerve under study.

EFS is monitored either automatically by the pressure of the heel on the ground, or by goniometric contact for the upper limb.

More developed programmes are in the experimental stage.

1.2. EFS by Implanted Electrodes

Nerve tissue tolerance to chronic implantations is a problem, which is still not completely resolved, even with platinum electrodes which are considered to have the best tolerance.

Peroneal nerve stimulation has already been used on a large scale. The method of collar electrodes developed at Ranchos Los Amigos Hospital by McNeal, has proved its efficiency; all the nerve structures are included in the collar, The Ljubljana implant developed by Jeglic is placed close to the nerve, according to the result of initial stimulation. Thus, it is possible to have quite a selective stimulation of the desired funiculi. McNeal has recently reported the use of platinum electrodes embedded in silicone and wrapped around the femoral nerve. Local tolerance of tissues appears to be excellent (control after 6 years) unless the electrode is subjected to minimal displacements during walking.

Muscle fibre changes following stimulation have been described by many: McNeal observed that excessive stimulation could induce metabolic alterations in skeletal muscle which did not appear when the stimulated muscle was tenotomized beforehand.

The observations suggest that "the pattern of electrical stimulation was less important than the conditions of the contraction process itself".

"Although a phasic pattern of stimulation was utilized, the type of conversion that occurred was determined not only by the pattern of stimulation, but rather by the physical conditions of contraction. If the muscle contracted isometrically, at a lengthened position and again resistance, stimulation resulted in an increased proportion of both type I and II fibers. If on the other hand the muscle contracted isotonically at a shortened length and with lesser resistance, type I fibers decreased proportionally in number and size" (McNeal 1976).

"Self regulatory mechanism within the myofiber itself are important."

1.3. EFS of the Spinal Cord

A number of stimulators have been implanted on the posterior column of the spinal cord for intractable pain. In recalling the facilitatory effect of painful stimuli on spasticity, we can infer that the reduction of pain following posterior column stimulation would simultaneously reduce spasticity. This was observed by Cook and Weinstein[15] (1973) in five patients with spastic painful paraplegia (flexion type), due to disseminated sclerosis. The same result was observed by Siegfried (1975) in two patients. Since then, we have operated on 3 patients with the same condition, but after an initial good result, all 3 patients relapsed.

2. Clinical Effect of EFS

In the hemiplegic spastic patient, whatever the etiology, the effect of EFS is immediately apparent, because in the action of walking, as soon as the heel is raised to start the swing phase of gait, stimulation occurs; the foot is dorsally flexed and stimulation will cease only when the heel again reaches the ground and switches out the SEF.

Relaxation of antagonist muscles is obtained with a decrease of hyperactive tendon reflexes (Fig. 11 and 12).

After repetitive stimulation, the whole function of the limb is usually improved; relaxation of the soleus muscle could last for several days and the strength of the dorsiflexors of the foot remain improved, the patient being able to walk without a stick. According to Gracanin, 5 per cent of the patients having used the Ljubljana stimulator for a longer period of time do not need the device any longer.

Results are not so clear cut when EFS is used for correction of spasticity in the upper limb. The patient can perform extension movements and if function of the flexor muscles is partially preserved, he may be able to hold objects; but this is not always obtained at once, and in many cases will appear only after long term, EFS so spasticity of flexors will clear and the patient's extensors become active. Quality of results is directly due to facilitation of minimal activity provided such in present.

3. Pathophysiology of EFS

F. Gracanin *et al.* have made[40] a very complete study of their group of patients submitted to long term EFS (1972). Inotation from this work helps in the understanding of neurophysiological problems which are not an every day preoccupation for neurosurgeons.

"At the beginning of stimulation, what can be termed efferent functional electrical stimulation, produces a rough contraction. Because of the lower threshold of the afferent nervous fibers in such a stimulation . . . there also exist artificial sensory inflows, via I a fibers, via low threshold cutaneous afferent fibers and via afferent fibers of the flexion reflex . . . directly impinging upon the spinal motoneurones."

"Stimulation of the peroneal nerve with intensity which does not cause the motor response in peroneal muscles, might have an inhibitory effect on the reflex response of the antagonist soleus muscle, such as the Hoffmann reflex, persisting sometime after the conditioning stimulus. This inhibitory effect may be exerted on uncontrolled motor activity such as clonus" (Figs. 11–12).

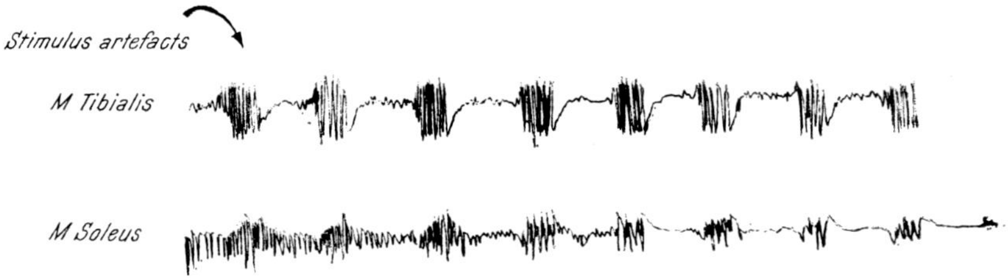

Fig. 11. In a patient with well marked clonus, complete inhibition during repeated stimulation was achieved (after Gracanin)

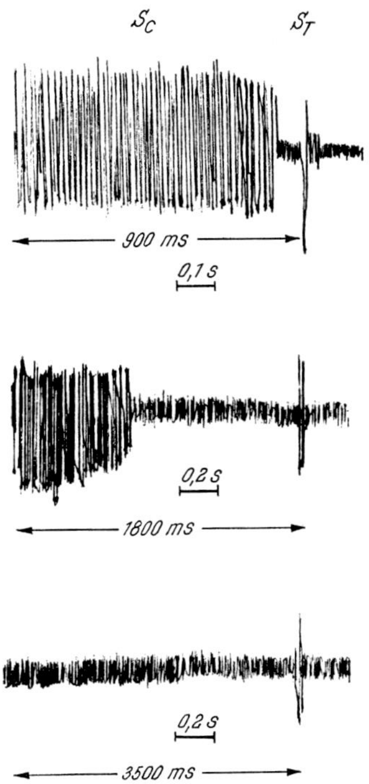

Fig. 12. Long-term inhibition of the H-reflex of the soleus muscle during electrical stimulation of the peroneal nerve at the level of the head of the fibula. The conditioning test interval is 900, 1800 and 3500 m/sec (after Gracanin)

"Long term stimulation has an effect on the organization of the reflex motor activity and brings restoration of the reciprocal motor activity pattrens in automatic movements such as gait."

"Long term depression is attributed to the inhibitory action of the interneural system. Investigations carried out by Eccles; Evans, Curtis and Eccles, showed that presynaptic mechanisms were responsible for such strong and long term changes."

And Gracanin concluded: "EFS is used to consciously engage propioceptive and musculocutaneous mechanism having a strong effect on the organization of reflex activity at various levels of the central nervous system. So far, the organization of the reflex motor activity and movements is integrated at the level of the spinal cord."

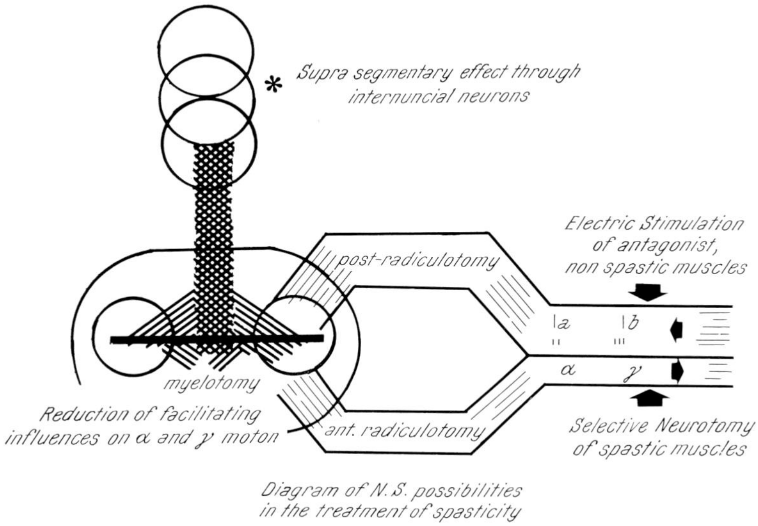

Fig. 13. Diagram of N. S. possibilities in the treatment of spasticity

VI. Indications for Treatment

There is no miracle operation which specifically reduces spasticity and reestablishes the normal balance of tone (Fig. 13).

The numerous functional neurosurgical possibilities given here, propose to reduce the facilitory influences on the alpha neurone in very different ways, but all use the same common physiological principles:

1. Action on the spastic agonist muscles to liberate the tonus of the antagonist muscles (peripheral neurotomies, posterior radiculotomies of the spastic sectors); stimulation of the non spastic agonists, to suppress the spasticity of the spastic antagonists. The segmentary effect is not identical but it is comparable.

2. Functional reorganization which acts on the whole spinal cord (suprasegmentary effect). It is at the same time a function of the extent of the operated area, the quantity of the facilitatory influxes which are reduced and the length and quality of the reeducation, either classic or with the help of the FES which will be applied afterwards. This is the rehabilitation programme to develop new motor patterns, in which NS must be inte-

grated at the right time. "When" and "what to do" must be studied with all the neurological factors concerned:

The possibility of functional reeducation must be respected for as long as it remains effective.

Voluntary motor activity, often hidden by the spasticity must now be correctly assessed.

Surgery must have a good chance of improving functional aptitude with no risk of increased deficit.

1. The Spastic Child

Infantile spastic hemiplegia—infantile spastic quadriplegia . . .

In the child the characteristic of motor and tonic equilibrium is its evolution. The child goes through successive stages where the clinical picture changes; we have seen that an early (1 year) and regular reeducation limits, but does not prevent, the appearance of pathological spastic motor patterns which are often complicated by abnormal movements.

The skeletal growth articular development, are directly influenced by spasticity which in severe form can create irreversible orthopaedic disorders. The child's I.Q. and psychological attitude will permit one to judge the future collaboration of the child, or its inertia, a determinant element of later reeducation.

These elements fix the age at which neurosurgery can be considered, when indicated, as from 6 to 7 years old.

The spastic type—"Little's disease"—usually has several handicapped sectors: hip flexion with lumbar hyperlordosis, thigh adduction and equinovarus.

Cessation of functional progress, poorly tolerated applicances, dangerous deformation of the hip and of the feet, leave no other alternative to articular and cutaneous complications, than operation.

There is a good prognosis for those children with a high I.Q., for those who kept voluntary motor activity, at least partially as, judged by a Procaïne subarachnoidal test.

The technique best adapted to these cases is sectorial posterior radiculotomy, which aims at suppressing the spasticity of the handicapped sectors without disturbing the tonal balance of the antigravity muscles, and respecting sphincter innervation.

We have seen that it is possible by keeping 1/5 of the rootlets radicelles in the sectors to be treated, so as to avoid a notable sensory deficit.

Reeducation is necessarily prolonged. There is an initial loss of functional level which from the very first analysis indicates a decrease in spasticity.

Reeducation will last at least 6 months in a specialized centre, where the actions of straightening up and standing erect are undertaken successively, before walking itself is embarked upon.

In favourable cases, the newly acquired motor balance permits walking with light appliances, or without appliances, often without a cane.

In more serious cases, the new muscular balance is accompanied by a new articular balance and this corrects subluxations. With time the vertebral balance improves, tolerance of appliances improves, and eventually light corrective appliances can be used.

The effect of spasticity on the upper limbs, especially where hands are concerned, is constant but less notable.

Spasticity limited to minor forms of Little's syndrome may be the subject of selective neurotomies, according to the analytic evaluation of the handicapped sector; most often it involves neurotomy of the soleus, of the posterior tibialis and sometimes the toe flexors. For this reeducation is easy and rapid, the motor patterns not being disturbed.

Spasticity of the upper limb rarely justifies operation. As for the lower limb, it is the existence of a handicapping spasticity, which can justify sectorial posterior radiculotomy.

The dystonic and dyskinetic syndromes and the chronic athetoses, cannot usefully benefit from the preceding operations which only act on spasticity; but they frequently justify different functional neurosurgery: concerning with the posterior nucleus of the thalamus, the subthalamic field of Forel etc. . . . This is a different problem and does not come into the framework of this study.

2. Spastic Hemiplegia

The handicap of hemiplegia is not limited to spasticity, but if marked it can become by its importance an obstacle to reeducation, the dilemma being either to continue the reeducation risking an aggravation of spasticity; or to stop the reeducation and to lose the benefit already obtained; the depressive reactions following such a decision may be imagined.

In the lower limb, spasticity of the quadriceps keeps the knee in extension, the dorsi-flexion of the foot is paralysed and the spasticity in adduction flexion makes the act of step movement difficult with unsteady pressure of the foot to the ground.

To add to these disorders, pain is often very acute with an obsessional tone.

In the present state of therapeutic endeavor we consider the problem in two stages, the first being confined to functional electrical stimulation, the second to actual neuro-surgical operation.

1. The FES of the external popliteal sciatic nerve has its place from the 6th up to the 12th month. We have seen the results: direct motor effect on the dorsi-flexion of the foot, indirect effect on the reduction of the contracture of the antagonists.

The extent of the stimulations, initially 15 mns three times a day is eventually modified in proportion to the results; the initial trial must continue for about 15 days, the patient then deciding, according to the results obtained, wheher or not to continue the treatment.

With favourable response motor progress and reduction of spasticity permits the stimulations to be spaced further apart, and in a small number of cases, to cease completely, while retaining the initial functional benefit.

Selection of the patients can be made in relation to the initial neuro-physiological examination, but it can more easily be made from observation of the results obtained during the trial period of the first 15 days of treatment.

2. Selective Neurotomies can be considered after the first year. At this stage the medical situation is generally stabilized and the patient makes no further progress, whereas the reduction of spasticity permits a new start reeducation.

The effect of Selective Neurotomies, especially in the foot and toe flexors, is immediate, 4 elements are usually observed:

1. Disappearance of pain.
2. Cessation of jerking movements of the foot.
3. Better pressure on the ground due to the reduction of tonus in the dorsi-flexion muscles.
4. Reduction of spasticity of the quadriceps.

After a few days the patient can resume his reeducation, he can in future bend the knee, and press the foot solidly to the ground.

Recurrences do exist, they are above all the result of insufficient surgery, too limited in area or in the choice of the muscles treated.

3. The Spastic Hand of Hemiplegics

The spastic hand of hemiplegics is very characteristic and can arise in very many situations; a major sensory-motor lesion, such as one sees after hemispherectomy, or after massive hemispheric lesions, will completely suppress its role as stereotatic analyser and finely balanced tool.

An isolated pyramidal tract lesion, will be less handicapping and allow better results in reeducation.

For the patient who does not accept his handicap, the unaesthetic appearance of the hand, and the accompanying painful phenomena, it is possible to obtain tonic reequilibration, and reduction of pain, without any noticeable functional improvement.

The most effective treatment is a sectorial radiculotomy aimed at reducing flexor spasticity of the wrist and fingers. It is easier to programme than in the lower limbs, because of the small number of posterior roots and their anatomical disposition.

Per-operative stimulation permits mapping of those rootlets to be cut those serving flexion of the wrist and fingers, and those to be preserved, subserving the extensors.

The hand thus recovers a position approaching that of the physiological position, unless retraction has already developed. Pain is favourably influenced often signalled as this is the most important benefit of the operation.

Spastic hands with incomplete sensory-motor deficits, above all if they are accompanied by painful phenomena, can benefit from either a posterior rootlet section as of Sindou type, or a sectorial radiculotomy for the spastic muscular groups. The future is promising, although experience in this field is limited so far.

4. *Spastic Paraplegics*

We must distinguish between spasticity in extension with exaggeration of tonic stretch reflexs and spasticity in flexion where the defence reflexes released by peripheral stimulation are dominant.

4.1. Spasticity in Extension

The moment when SP is established as a handicapping element varies: it is early and intense if reeducation treatment has been badly directed; on the other hand it can happen unexpectedly, even very late after a period when the tonal balance appeared to be stabilized.

It is associated with spasmodic contractions which impede sitting in an armchair; it resists drugs and reduces appliance toleration, even at times hygienic care and transfer from chair to bed becomes impossible.

In these cases, as for the spastic child, the topography and the importance of the spasticity decide what choice will be made.

"Low spasticity" localized in the foot and toe flexors, demands solely peripheral selective neurotomies.

Complicated spasticity where the position of the hips in flexion-adduction dominates, or where there is also a spastic equinus often with irregular jerkings, justifies sectorial posterior radiculotomy.

Reeducation then helps functional progress, improves tolerance to appliances and has a direct action on the bladder hypertonus.

The initial results are not linked to the etiology of paraplegia, but to the specific character of true spasticity by exaggeration of the stretch reflex.

Late results do not exclude recurrences, which are in general limited and due to evolution of degenerative illnesses, operations to too restricted an area, or to increased noxious impulses from complications such as pressure sores, bladder infections and depressive attitudes.

4.2. The Spasticity Type in Flexion

In this spasticity all the osteo-tendinous reflexes have disappeared, there is no longer exaggeration of stretch reflexes, but a contracture in flexion, which exists at rest and increases in response to all external stimulation.

In order to judge the existance of fibrous retractions frequent at this stage, contracture is relaxed by root anaesthesia.

The spinal cord pathology is diffuse and often progressive (degenerative illnesses).

Surgery aiming to reduce the harmful facilitatory influences is not always effective (posterior radiculotomy); peripheral surgery too limited (neurotomy).

We prefer large anterior radiculotomies from L 1 to S 1 bilaterally. These bedridden patients, often cachectic, with large pressure sores, have, a surprising tolerance. These operations obtain good results in that pressure sores heal and deformities may be orthopaedically corrected. Bladder function is not altered.

We have no experience of myelotomies covering large areas as have Laitinen and Benedetti who have had excellent results; but we have some reserve as to the risk of aggravation of bladder disorders.

To end this chapter, we shall classify the indications for operation according to the results desired:

5. Indications

5.1. Indications for Functional Improvement

This relates to localized handicapping spasticity for which the technique varies according to the topography of the disorders. These are the very frequent indications for spasticity which dominates in a localized muscular group giving way to a specific disorder, in example "equinism of the foot, flexion adduction of the hip", etc. According to the localization of handicap, EFS, peripheral neurotomy or occasionally sectorial radiculotomy may be proposed. Wearing of appliances is usually either simplified or suppressed.

5.2. Indications for Articular Protection

These relate to the spasticity which is dangerous for articular equilibrium: subluxations of the hip, genu recurvatum, and valgus flat foot. In particular, it relates to intractable spasticity, for which limited surgery is insufficient and for which sectorial posterior radiculotomy is necessary.

5.3. Indications for Comfort

These relate particularly to intractable spasticity that resists medical treatment (severe spasticity in bedridden patients, spasticity in flexion) etc., corresponding to unfavourable cases, either to very progressive degenerative patients, or to patients showing serious complications at an early stage: serious bladder disorders, pressure sores, peri-articular ossification etc. . . . Surgery is performed to ease the posture in bed, the sitting position, hygienic care or pressure sores.

Only major operations are decided upon:

1. if spasticity in extension persists, posterior radiculotomy,
2. if paraplegia develops in flexion, anterior radiculotomy.

VII. Concluding Remarks

The appearance of spasticity, during cerebral nervous lesion, often presents the beginning of difficult reeducation problems.

Traditional means of prevention against spasticity (passive mobilization, posture, apparatus and orthopaedic surgery) seem uncomplete and in some way dangerous to us: as a matter of fact the setting of stretch reflex involves fighting reaction against apparatus with pain and articular deformation especially on feet:

We propose a different analysis of spasticity leading to a new treatment:

the "handicapping spasticity" only must be reduced contrary to the "useful spasticity" which must be preserved (standing up and walking).

The analytical clinical examination has to assess active muscular power, spasticity, functional possibilities, and determines the surgical treatment:

The object of this one is:

1. Orthopaedic prevention: balancing again agonist and antagonist muscles of threatened joints.

2. Functional improvement: when spasticity obstructs useful voluntary movement.

3. Comfort indication: so that apparatus tolerance got better.

Besides total surgical treatments of spasticity (myelotomy, dentatectomy pulvinarolysis, wide rhizotomy), we propose two different sorts of selective operation: attacking only muscular sectors with handicapping spasticity: sectorial posterior rhizotomy (SPR) and selective ramicellar neurotomy (SRN).

Peroperative stimulation and testing enable us to establish a mapping of the group of rootlets and nervous fascicules.

These sectorial techniques decrease the failure rate of the other techniques and even allow a functional improvement for spastic patients with stable level of reeducation.

Such operations need precise indications to be successful (cerebral palsy, Little scheme, spastic paraplegia).

The electrical functional stimulation used as complementary of sectorial surgical technique leads to a new therapeutic way.

References

1. Al-Moods, W. S., *et al.*, 1973: Longterm stimulation of cat fast twitch skeletal muscle. Nature *244*, 225—227.
2. Ashby, P., Verrier, M., Lightfoot, E., 1974: Segmental reflex pathways in spinal shock and spinal spasticity in man. J. Neurol. Neurosurg. Psychiat. *37*, 1352—1360.
3. Barker, D., 1968: L'innervation motrice des muscles striés. Actual. Neurophysiol. *8*, 23—71.
4. Benedetti, A., Carbonin, C., 1977: Résultats de la myelotomie lombaire dans les paraplégies spastiques avec contractions musculaires (observations préliminaires chez 12 malades). Neurochirurgie *23*, 347—353.
5. Bennett, A. H., 1888: Brain *10*, 289.
6. Benezech, J., 1975: Etude couplée des potentiels évoqués et du réflexe d'Hoffmann chez les traumatisés médullaires. Thèse médecine Montpellier.
7. Bischof, W., 1952: Die longitudinale Myelotomie, erstmalig zervikal durchgeführt. Zbl. Neurochir. *12*, 205—210.
8. Bischof, W., 1967: Zur dorsalen longitudinalen Myelotomie. Zbl. Neurochir. *28*, 123—126.
9. Bobath, K., Bobath, B., 1957: Control of motor function in the treatment of cerebral palsy. Physiotherapy *43*, 295.
10. Brondgeest, P. J., 1860: De tono musculorum voluntati sibidorum Hool. Breit. anat. Physiol. Wiss. Quoted by Fulton, J. F., 1926.
11. Cadilhac, J., Benezech, J., Georgesco, M., 1975: Etudes des potentiels évoqués et du réflexe d'Hoffmann dans les lésions traumatiques de la moelle. Revue d'EEG et Neuro Physiologie clinique *5*, 418.

12. Cadilhac, J., 1967: Les troubles expérimentaux du tonus musculaire. In: Girard, P. G., Pellet, H., pp. 516—529, Médecine Expérimentale, 1 vol. 587 pp. Paris: Masson.
13. Cajal (Ramon Y.) S., 1901: Histologie du système nerveux, *I*, 986 p. Paris: Maloine.
14. Collins, W., Nulsen, P., Randt, C., 1960: Relation of peripheral nerve fiber size and sensation in man. Arch. Neurol. *3*, 381—385.
15. Cook, A. W., Weinstein, S. P., 1973: Chronic dorsal stimulation in multiple sclerosis. Preliminary report. New York State J. Med. *73*, 2868—2872.
16. Cooper, I. S., 1971: Motor functions of the thalamus with recent observations concerning the role of the pulvinar Int. J. Neurol. *8*, 238—259.
17. Cooper, I. S., Amin, I., Chandra, R., 1973: A surgical investigation of the clinical physiology of the LP pulvinar complex in man. J. Neurol. Sci. *18*, 89—110.
18. Delmas-Marsalet, P., van Bogaert, L., 1935: Sur un cas de myoclonies rythmiques continues déterminées par une intervention chirurgicale sur le tronc cérébral. Revue Neurol. *64*, 728.
19. Delwaide, P. J., 1973: Human monosynaptic reflexes and presynaptic inhibition. In: New Developments in E. M. G. and Clinical Neurophysiology, *2*, 67—84. J. E. Desmedt, édit. Basel: Karger.
20. Desmedt, J. E., Noel, P., 1973: Average cerebral evoked potentials in the evaluation of lesions of the sensory nerves and of the central somatocensory pathway. In: New Developments in E. M. G. and Clinical Neurophysiology, *2*, 352—371. J. E. Desmedt, édit. Basel: Karger.
21. Dimitrijevic, M. R., Gracanin, F., 1967: Control of release phenomena in hemiplegics by means of afferent electrical stimulation. International Meeting on Electromyography, Glasgow. Electroenceph. Clin. Neurosphysiol. *25*, 395.
22. Dimitrijevic, W. R., Nathan, P. M., 1967, 1968: Studies of spasticity in man:
1. Some features of spasticity. Brain *90*, 1—30.
2. Analysis of strech reflex in spasticity. Brain *90*, 333—358.
3. Analysis of reflex activity evoked by noxious cutaneous stimulation. Brain *91*, 349—368.
23. Djalali, F., 1970: Relations neurophysiologiques brachio-lombaires chez le chat spinal. Thèse de doctorat es-Sciences Naturelles, Aix-Marseille I, C. N. R. S. 4.674 A. O., dactylo. 150 P.
24. Eccles, J. C., 1957: The physiology of nerve cells, p. 270. Baltimore: The Johns Hopkins Press.
25. Eccles, J. C., 1964: The physiology of synapses, pp. 220—238. Berlin-Heidelberg-New York: Springer.
26. Eccles, J. C., 1969: The inhibitory pathways of the central nervous system. The Sherrington lectures IX. Springfield, Ill.: Ch. C Thomas.
27. Feld, M., Pecker, J., 1951: Essais de cordotomie postérieure dans les paraplégies spasmodiques. Application au syndrome paraplégique de Little. Sté. Neurochir. langue française *85*, 542—548.
28. Foerster, O., 1908: Über eine neue operative Methode der Behandlung spastischer Lähmungen mittels Resektion hinterer Rückenmarkswurzeln. Z. Ortop. Chir. *22*, 203.
29. Foerster, O., 1913: On the indications and results of the excision of posterior spinal nerve roots in men. Surg. Gynec. Obstet. *16*, 463—474.
30. Fraioli, B., 1973: Spasticita: problemi fisiopatologici, clinici e terapeutici. Riv. Neurol. *43*, 196—228.
31. Fraioli, B., Guidetti, B., 1975: Effects of stereotactic lesions of the pulvinar and lateralis posterior nucleus on intractable pain and dyskinetic syndromes of man. Appl. Neurophys. *38*, 23—30.
32. Fraioli, B., Guidetti, B., 1977: Effects of the stereotactic lesion of the dentate nucleus of the cerebellum in man. Appl. Neurophys. *38*, 81—90.

33. Fraioli, B., Guidetti, B., 1975: La rizotomia posteriore parziale ed una nuova tecnica, la radicolotomia posteriore parziale, nel trattamento della spasticita tonica. Riv. Pat. Nerv. Ment. *96*, 65—81.
34. Fraioli, B., Guidetti, B., La Torre, E., 1972: La dentalolisi stereotassica nel trattamento della spasticita e delle discinesie. Gazz. San. *78*, 297.
35. Fulton, J. F., 1926: Muscular contraction and the reflex control of movement, p. 644. Baltimore: Williams & Wilkins Comp. 1926.
36. Fuxe, K., 1965: Evidence for the existence of monoamine containing neurons in the central nervous system. IV. Distribution of monoamine terminals in the central nervous system. Acta Physiol. Scand. 64 supp., *247*, 39—85.
37. Granit, R., 1955, 1956: Receptors and sensory perception. A discussion of aims, means and results of electrophysiological research into the process of reception. New Haven: Yale Univ. Press. 1955. Ibid. J. Physiol. (Lond.) *131*, 32.
38. Gracanin, F. T., *et al.*, 1967: Evaluation of use of functional electronic peroneal brace in hemiparetic patients. External Control of human extremities. Intern. Symposium Dubrovnik 1966.
39. Gracanin, F., Grobelnik, J., 1968: Clinical and technical evaluation of the Ljubljana functional electronic peroneal brace. Proceeding of the Symposium on electronics in Medicine, Ljubljana, *9*, 12.
40. Gracanin, F., 1972: Use of functional stimulation in rehabilitation of hemiplegic patients, 109 p. The Institute of the SR slovenia for rehabilitation of the disabled. Ljubljana, Yugoslavia.
41. Gros, C., Privat, J. M., Benezech, J., Frerebeau, P., 1976: Sectorial posterior rhizotomy, a new technique of surgical treatment for spasticity. Acta Neurochir. (Wien) *35*, 181—195.
42. Gros, C., Ouaknine, G., Vlahovitch, B., Frerebeau, Ph., 1967: La radicotomie sélective postérieure dans le traitement neurochirurgical de l'hypertonie pyramidale. Neuro-chirurgie *13*, 505—518.
43. Gros, C., Frerebeau, Ph., Kuhner, A., Perez-Dominguez, E., Privat, J. M., 1973: Technical modification in the Foerster operation. Selective posterior lumbar roots section. The results of 18 years of practice. International Congress of Neuro-Surgery, Tokyo, october 1973.
44. Gros, C., Frerebeau, Ph., Privat, J. M., Perez-Dominguez, E., Bazin, M., 1976: Chirurgie stéréotaxique dans les dystonies et dyskinésies non parkinsoniennes. A propos d'une série personnelle de 48 cas. Neuro-chirurgie *22*, No. 6, 539—552.
45. Gros, C., *et al.*, 1977: Table ronde sur la chirurgie de la spasticité. Société Française de Neurochirurgie. Neuro-chirurgie *23*, 316—388.
46. Grossiord, A., Tardieu, C., Lacert, Ph., 1975: Approche électrologique de la réflectivité des paraplégiques. Ann. Méd. Physique *18*, 245—254.
47. Guidetti, B., Fraioli, B., 1976: Problèmes cliniques et possibilités neurochirurgicales actuelles dans les syndromes dyskinétiques. Neuro-chirurgie *22*, 552—561.
48. Guidetti, B., Fraioli, B., Neurosurgical treatment of spasticity and dyskinesias Acta Neurochir. (in press).
49. Guth, L., *et al.*, 1972: Physiological and histo-chemical properties of the soleus muscle after denervation of its antagonists. Exp. Neurol. *36*, 463—471.
50. Hagbarth, K. E., Eklund, G., 1966: Motor effect of vibratory muscle stimuli in man. In 33 Proceeding of the first Nobel Symposium Stockholm, pp. 177, 186. R. Granit, ed. Stockholm: Almquist et Wiksell. 1966.
51. Hagbarth, K. E., 1967: Vibration of muscles in the cerebral palsied children. Personal communication.
52. Heimburger, R. F., *et al.*, 1973: Cervical posterior rhizotomy for reducing spasticity in cerebral palsy. J. Neurosurg. *39*, 30—34.
53. Heimburger, R. F., 1968: Stereotaxic destruction of the human dentate nucleus. Confin. Neurol. *26*, 358—396.
54. Held, J. P., Pierrot-Deseilligny, E., 1969: Rééducation motrice des affectations neurologiques, 200 p. Paris: Baillière, ed.

55. Herman, R., 1970: The myototic reflex; clinico-physiological aspects of spasticity and contracture. Brain *93*, 273—312.
56. Jansen, J., 1954: Efferent cerebellar connections. In: Jansen, J., Brodal, A. (eds.), Johan Grundt Traum (publ.). Aspects of cerebellar anatomy. *I*, 189.
57. Jansen, J. K. S., 1962: Spasticity. Functional aspects. Acta Neurol. Scand. *38*, sup. 3, 41—51.
58. Jeglic, A., *et al.*, 1966, 1967: Electrical stimulation of skeletal muscles by directly powered implanted radio frequency receivers. Proceeding of International Symposium on External control of Human Extremities, pp. 42, 53, Dubrovnik 1966, and Yugoslavian Conference for electronics and automation, Beograd 1967.
59. Kanaka, T. S., Balasubramanian, V., 1974: Stereotaxic pulvinotomy for cerebral palsy. Proc. Inst. Neurol. Madras *4*, 58—62.
60. Keats, S., 1957: Combined adductor-gracilis tenotomy and selective obturator-nerve resection for the correction of adduction deformity of the hips in children with cerebral palsy. J. Bone and Joint Surg. *39 A*, 1087—1090.
61. Krayenbühl, H., Siegfried, J., 1969: La Chirurgie stéréotaxique du noyau dentelé dans le traitement des hyperkinésies et des états spastiques. Neuro-chir. (Paris) *15*, 51.
62. Laitinen, L., Singounas, E., 1971: Longitudinal myelotomy in the treatment of spasticity of the legs. J. Neurosurg. *35*, 536—540.
63. Levine, M. G., Knott, Kabat, 1952: Relation of spasticity by electrical stimulation of antagonist muscles. Arch. Phys. Med. *33*, 668—673.
64. Liberson, W. T., Holmquest, H., Scot, D., Dow, M., 1961: Functional electrotherapy: stimulation of the peroneal nerve synchronized with the swing phase of the gait of hemiplegic patients. Arch. Phys. Med. 42.
65. Liberson, W. T., 1965: Experiment concerning reciprocal inhibition of antagonists elicited by electrical stimulation of agonists in a normal individual. Amer. J. Phys. Med. *36*, 306—308.
66. Liljestrand, G., Magnus, R., 1919: Pflüg. Arch. ges. Physiol. *176*, 168.
67. Lundberg, A., 1967: Supraspinal control of transmission in spinal reflex pathways. In: Recent Advance in Clinical Neurophysiology. Electroenceph. clin. Neurophysiol., sup. *25*, 35—46.
68. Matthews, P. C. B., Rushworth, G., 1956: J. Physiol. (Lond.) *131*, 30.
69. Matthews, P. B. C., 1972: Mammalian muscle receptors and their central action, 612 p. London: E. Arnold. 1972.
70. Maury, M., Audic, B., Guillaumat, M., Francois, N., 1975: L'évolution de la spasticité dans le centre de paraplégiques adultes hommes. Ann. Méd. Physique *18*, 567—570.
71. McCarty, C. S., Kiefer, E. J., 1949: Thoracic lumbar and sacral spinal cordectomy. Proc. Staff. Meet. Mayo Clin. *24*, 108.
72. McNeal, D. R., Wilemon, W. K., 1969: Treatment of spasticity through functional electrical stimulation. Neuroelectric conference San Francisco, February.
73. McNeal, D. R., 1973: Peripheral nerve stimulation: Superficial and implanted in fields WS red.: Neural organization and its relevance to prosthetics, pp. 77—100. New York: Intercontinental Medical Book Corp.
74. McNeal, D., Munsat, Th., Waters, R., 1976: Effects of nerve stimulation on human muscle. Arch. Neurol. *33*, 606—617.
75. Melzack, R., Wall, P., 1965: Pain mechanisms: a new theory. Science *150*, 971—979.
76. Mendell, L., Wall, P., 1965: Responses of single dorsal cord cells of peripheral cutaneous unmyelinated fibers. Nature *206*, 97—99.
77. Milani Comparetti, A., 1965: Spasticity versus patterned postural and motor behaviour of spastics. Europa Medicophysica I, 3, I, 7.
78. Moyes, P. D., 1969: Longitudinal myelotomy for spasticity. J. Neurosurg. *31*, 615—619.
79. Monro, D., 1945: The rehabilitation of patients totally paralysed below waist: anterior rhizotomy for spastic paraplegia. New Engl. J. Med. *233*, 456—461.

80. Nashold, B. S., Slaughter, D. G., 1969: Effects of stimulating of destroying the deep cerebellar regions in man. J. Neurosurg. *31*, 172.
81. Ouaknine, G., 1965: La radicotomie sélective postérieure dans le traitement de l'hypertonie pyramidale, 98 p. Thèse Med., Montpellier.
82. Paillard, J., 1955: Réflexes et régulations d'origine proprioceptive chez l'homme. Thèse Sciences.
83. Perot, Pl., 1973: The clinical use of somatosensory evoked potentials in spinal cord injury. Clin. Neurosurg. *20*, 367—381.
84. Pette, D., *et al.*, 1973: Effects of long-term electrical stimulation on some contractile and metabolic characteristics of fast rabbit muscles. Pflüg. Arch. ges. Physiol. *338*, 257—272.
85. Phelps, W. M., 1951: Treatment of paralytic disorders exclusive of poliomyelitis: In: Baucroft, F. W., Marble, H. C., Surgical treatment of the motor-skeletal system. Philadelphia: J. B. Lippincott Co.
86. Pierrot-Desseilligny, E., 1969: Le réflexe "H", son intéret pour l'exploration fonctionelle du système nerveux. Presse Médicale *77*, 4—10.
87. Pierrot-Desseilligny, F., Bussel, B., Morin, C., 1973: Supraspinal control of the changes induced in H-reflex by cutaneous stimulation as studied in normal and spastic man. In: New Developments in E. M. G. and clinical Neurophysiology, Vol. 2, pp. 67—84. J. E. Desmedt, édit. Basel: Karger.
88. Pollock, L. J., Davis, L. E., 1923, 1930, 1931: Arch. Neurol. Psychiat. Chicago *10*, 391; Ibid., *23*, 303. Amer. J. Physiol. *98*, 47.
89. Pourpre, M. H., 1960: Traitement neurochirurgical des contractures chez les paraplégiques post-traumatiques. Neurochirurgie *6*, 229—236.
90. Privat, J. M., 1976: La radicotomie postérieure sectorielle. Communication présentée à la table ronde sur la chirurgie de la spasticité. Société Française de Neurochirurgie. Les Arcs (cf. Ref. 30).
91. Privat, J. M., Benezech, J., Frerebeau, Ph., Gros, C., 1976: Sectorial posterior rhizotomy; a new technique of surgical treatment of spasticity. Ve European Neurosurgical Congress, Oxford, sept. 1975. Acta Neurochir. (Wien) *35*, 181—195.
92. Privat, Ch., 1974: La radicotomie sélective postérieure dans le cadre de la rééducation fonctionnelle de l'hypertonie. Mémoire — Montpellier, 70 p.
93. Privat, Ch., Frerebeau, Ph., Privat, J. M., Gros, C., 1975: La radicotomie sélective postérieure dans le cadre de la rééducation fonctionnelle de l'hypertonie. Evolution de la notion de sélectivité III èmes entretiens de rééducation et de réadaptation fonctionnelles. Montpellier, Mars 1975. Cahiers Rééd., Réadapt. *10*, 229—236.
94. Riley, D. A., *et al.*, 1973: The effects of inactivity, programmed stimulation and denervation on the histochemistry of skeletal muscle fiber types. Exp. Neurol. *40*, 391—413.
95. Romanu, F. C. A., van der Meulen, J. P., 1967: Slow and fast muscle after crossinnervation: Enzymatic and physical changes. Arch. Neurol. *17*, 387—402.
96. Ralston, H., 1965: The organization of substantia gelatinosa Rolandi in the cat lumbo-sacral spinal cord. Zellforsch. *67*, 1—23.
97. Rondot, P., 1968: Etudes cliniques et physiopathologique des contractures. Rev. Neurol. *118*, 321—342.
98. Rushworth, G., 1960: Spasticity and rigidity: an experimental study and review. J. Neurol. Neurosurg. Psychiat. *23*, 97—117.
99. Sherrington, C. S., 1909: On plastic tonus and proprio ceptive reflexes. Quart. J. exp. physiol. *II*, 109—156.
100. Siegfried, J., 1971: Stereotaxic cerebellar surgery. Confin. Neurol. *33*, 350—358.
101. Siegfried, J., 1972: Stereotactic treatment of hypertonicity. In: Present limits of neurosurgery. I. Fusek and Z. Kunc, eds., I vol., pp. 549—550. Prague: Avicenum.
102. Siegfried, J., 1974: Methods and results in hyperkinesia and hypertonicity. In: Recent progress in neurological surgery. K. Sano and S. Ischii, eds., I vol., pp. 251—255. Amsterdam: Experta Medica; New York: American Elsevier.
103. Siegfried, J., 1977: Stereotactic pulvinarotomy in the treatment of intractable pain. Progress Neurol. Surg. Vol. 8, Part II, 104—113.

104. Siegfried, J., Verdie, J. C., Long term assessment of sterotactic dentatomy for spasticity. Acta Neurochir. (Wien) Suppl. 24, pp. 41—48.
105. Silver, C. M., Simon, S. D., 1959: Gastrocnemius muscle recession (Silfverskiold operation) for spastic-equinus deformity in cerebral palsy. J. Bone and Joint Surg. *41 A*, 1021—1028.
106. Silfverskiold, N., 1923—1924: Reduction of the uncrossed two-joint muscles of the leg. to one-joint muscles in spastic condition. Acta Chir. Scand. *56*, 315—322.
107. Sindou, M., 1972: Etude de la jonction radiculo-médullaire postérieure. La radicellotomie postérieure sélective dans la chirurgie de la douleur, 182 p. Thèse Med., Lyon.
108. Sindou, M., Fischer, G., Goutelle, A., Schott, B., Mansuy, L., 1974: La radicellotomie postérieure sélective dans le traitement des spasticités. Rev. Neurol. *b*, *130*, 201—216.
109. Steinberger, W. W., *et al.*, 1968: Maintenance of denervated rabbit muscle with direct electrostimulation. Arch. Phys. Med. Rehabil. *49*, 573—577.
110. Stoffel, A., 1912—1913: The treatment of spastic contracture. Am. J. Orthop. Surg. *10*, 611.
111. Szentagothai, I., 1974: Neuronal and synaptic arrangement in the substantia gelatinosa. J. Comp. Neurol. *122*, 219—239.
112. Tardieu, G., Got, G., Lespargot, A., 1975: Indications d'un nouveau type d'infiltrations au point moteur (Alcool à 96°). Ann. Méd. Physique *18*, 539—556.
113. Tardieu, G., 1962: Action des infiltrations d'alcool dilué sur diverses raideurs liées aux lésions cérébrales. Bull. et Mém. Soc. Méd. Hôp. de Paris *113*, 1, 7, 12.
114. Tardieu, G., Got, C., Lespargot, A., 1975: Indication d'un nouveau type d'infiltration au point moteur (alcool à 96°). Application clinique d'une étude expérimentale. Ann. Méd. Physique *18*, 539—557.
115. Tarlov, I. M., 1967: Rigidity in man due to spinal interneuron loss. Arch. Neurol. *16*, 536, 443.
116. Tönnis, W., Bischof, W., 1962: Ergebnisse der lumbalen Myelotomie nach Bischof. Zbl. Neurochir. *23*, 120—132.
117. Valbo, A. B., Hagbarth, K. E., 1973: Microelectrode recording from human peripheral nerves. In: New Developments in E. M. G. and Clinical Neurophysiology, *2*, 67—84. J. E. Desmedt, édit. Basel: Karger.
118. Vedel, J. D., 1973: Cortical control of dynamic and static gamma motoneuron activity. In: New Developments in E. M. G. and Clinical Neurophysiology, *3*, 126—135. J. E. Desmedt, édit. Basel: Karger.
119. Verdie, J. C., 1975: Le noyau dentelé. Données fondamentales. Analyse de 50 cas de dentatotomies stéréotaxiques, 178 p. Thèse med. Toulouse, Octobre.
120. Vodovnik, L., Dimitrijevic, M. R., Prevec, T., Logar, M., 1966: Electronic walking aids for patients with peroneal palsy. Wld. Electron. Inst. 4/2, 58.
121. Vodovnik, L., 1969: Stimulation of spastic extremities: some engineering considerations. Proceedings of the 8th Intern. conference on Medical and Biological Engineering, Chicago 1969.
122. Weaver, R. A., Landau, W. M., Higgins, J. P., *et al.*, 1963: Fusimotor function Part II. Evidence of fusimotor depression in human. Arch. Neurol. *9*, 127—132.
123. Wall, P., 1964: Presynaptic control of impulses at the first central synapse in the cutaneous pathway. In: Progress in brain research: physiology of spinal neurons, pp. 92—118. J. Eccles and J. Schade, eds. New York: Elsevier Publ. Co.
124. Walshe, F. M. R., 1924: Procaine injection for spasticity. Brain *47*, 159—172.
125. Yamada, S., Perot, L., Ducker, T. B.: Longitudinal myelotomy for control of mass spasms in paraplegia. 5th International Congress of Neurological Surgery, Tokyo 1973.

B. Technical Standards

Surgical Approaches to the Sphenoidal and Clival Areas

P. J. Derome and G. Guiot

In co-operation with

B. Georges, M. Porta, A. Visot, and S. Balagura

Service de Neurochirurgie, Hôpital Foch, Suresnes (France)

With 25 Figures

Contents

Introduction

The sphenoid occupies a central position within the head. Its intracranial surface forms part of the wall of the anterior, middle and posterior fossae, while its extracranial surface contributes to the posterior and superior borders of the nasal fossae.

The clivus, formed by the sphenoid and occipital bones, extends from the dorsum sellae to the anterior margin of the foramen magnum. In children, a cartilaginous plate is found at the sphenoid-occipital junction; this suture disappears in the adult, except on rare occasions. It is interesting to note that this synchondrosis may act as a barrier for some pathological conditions, *i.e.*, fibrous dysplasia, which remain limited to either of these bones.

A variety of pathological conditions may affect this area. There are many primary bone tumors of the base of the skull, *i.e.*, chondromas or chordomas. Other tumors result from secondary invasion of the bone, *i.e.*, meningiomas or nasopharyngeal neoplasms. Other lesions are not truly neoplastic, as is the case with fibrous dysplasia. Mucoceles of the sphenoid sinuses should be considered in the differential diagnosis of local pathology.

The special anatomical position of the sphenoidal-clival region lends itself to several, distinct, surgical approaches: lateral subtemporal, posterior occipital, transcervical, transoral, rhino-septal, and transbasal. The surgeon must choose the route that will permit the most complete removal of the lesion with minimal danger to the patient. Occasionally a change of the approach, or even a combination of various surgical approaches may be indicated to achieve tumor removal, decompression of the brain stem, and freeing of entrapped cranial nerves.

I. Intradural Approaches

Before considering the anterior approaches, which are the main topic of this paper, we will briefly discuss the more conventional posterior and lateral routes to the clival region. Together they offer a wide range of surgical choices.

a) Subtemporal Approach

This remains the most popular route to tumors of the upper clivus which often compress the brainstem. Intratumoral resection in the case of large lesions usually facilitates the procedure, which may be more difficult when working within the confines of smaller tumors. Large neoplasms which normally grow in a rostro-caudal direction displace cranial nerves laterally and basally. Section of the tentorium along the upper edge of the petrous bone and the superior petrosal sinus facilitates the procedure. Temporal lobe ischemia may result from the prolonged application of a retractor, and caution must be taken in its placement. Positioning of the patient supine with the head turned to one side allows spontaneous retraction of the temporal lobe not afforded by the half-sitting position often advocated. This factor should be considered when operating from the dominant temporal side.

b) Suboccipital Approach

This route affords access to the lower part of the clivus down to the foramen magnum. The patient is placed in the sitting position with the head rotated about 15 degrees to the side of the approach. The posterior fossa is exposed widely from the lateral bend of the transverse sinus to the midline, and below to the posterior ridge of the foramen magnum. Tumor resection is rendered difficult by the various cranial nerves interposed between surgeon and tumor. When the lesion extends caudally to the foramen magnum and the cervical spine, the vertebral arteries may be deflected backwards over the tumor surface. One can attempt total removal even in cases when the tumor lies in front of the brainstem. Intratumoral removal between the nerves often provides enough space to reach the opposite pole of the neoplasm. When hemodynamic conditions permit section of one vertebral artery, beyond the origin of the posterior inferior cerebellar artery, tumor dissection may be greatly facilitated (Figs. 1 a, b, c, d).

In cases involving the whole clival area, the lesion may be resected using the *subtemporal and suboccipital approaches in combination* (Fig. 2). A modified "hockey-stick" incision, curved over the temporal and straight over the occipital region, is made one centimeter behind the mastoid. The transverse sinus is dissected free and severed just before the drainage site of the vein of Labbé. The combined section of the transverse sinus and the tentorium allows for an ample supra and infra tentorial exposure (care must be taken that the patient has a patent contralateral sinus). The technical problems remain the same as for each individual approach, but one can often resect rather extensive tumors in the same surgical session.

These two surgical approaches are called for in cases of tumors situated behind the clivus. The exposure they give does not permit the neurosurgeon to resect a neoplastic process invading the bone on the basal midline. They permit an intradural resection, and, with the exception of some tumors involving the petrous bone, an extradural approach to the sphenoid and clivus is not possible.

II. Anterior Approaches

The sphenoidal-clival area may be approached from four different routes given the anatomy of the cranio-facial region, *i.e.*, transcervical, transoral, transsphenoidal, and transbasal. All converge at a different angle over the clival area.

a) Transcervical Approach

Such an approach was first described by Stevenson *et al.*[13] after the experimental work of White and Albin. A curvilinear, submandibular incision is made from the mastoid tip to the symphysis menti, with a "T" extension across the sternocleidomastoid to the level of C_6. The Axis and Atlas are exposed between the neck vessels and the trachea. The prebulbar dura, or as in the case of a chordoma, the arachnoid, can be reached by resection of the anterior arch of the Atlas, the odontoid, the lower part of the clivus, and the anterior rim of the foramen magnum.

The difficulties encountered in this surgical procedure are similar to those encountered in other anterior approaches, *i.e.*, the great depth of the operative field (though the problem is less when working with the aid of the

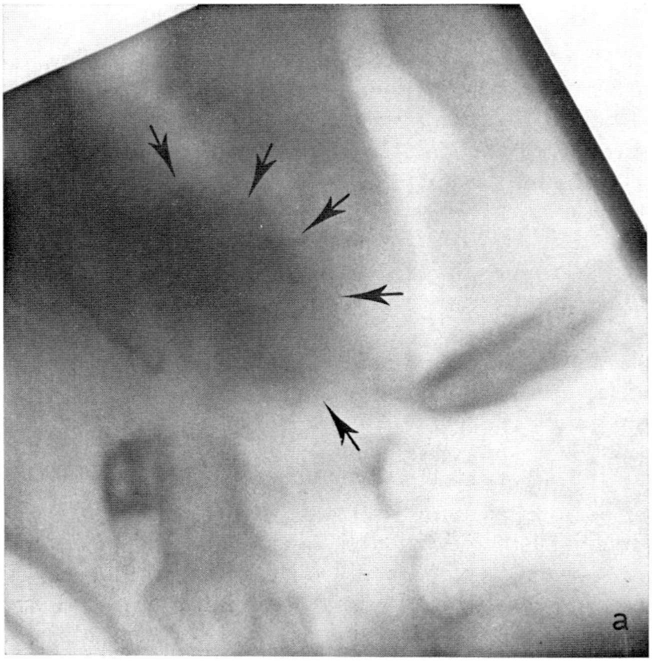

Fig. 1a

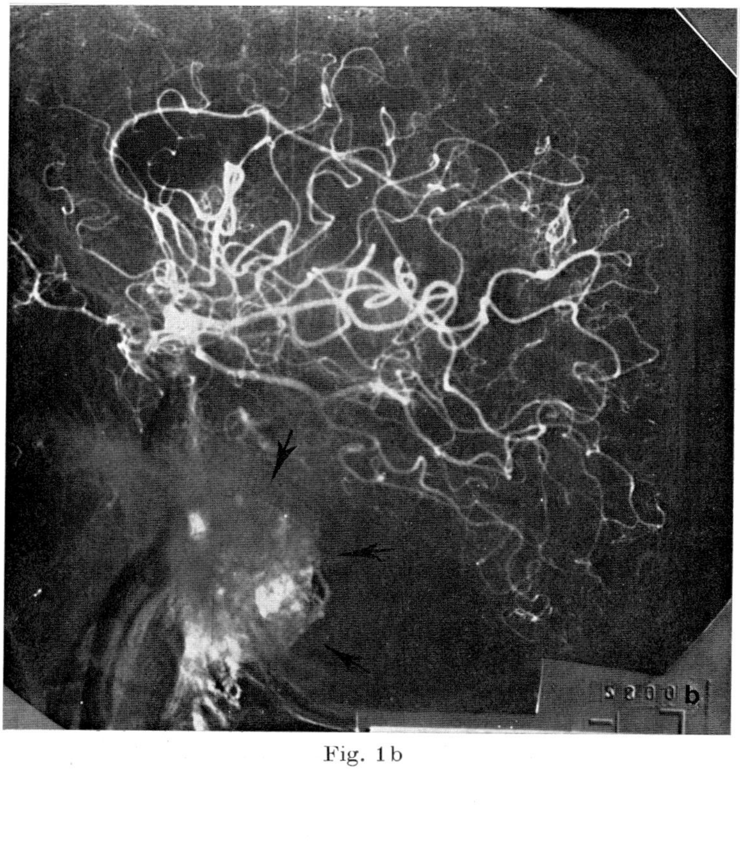

Fig. 1b

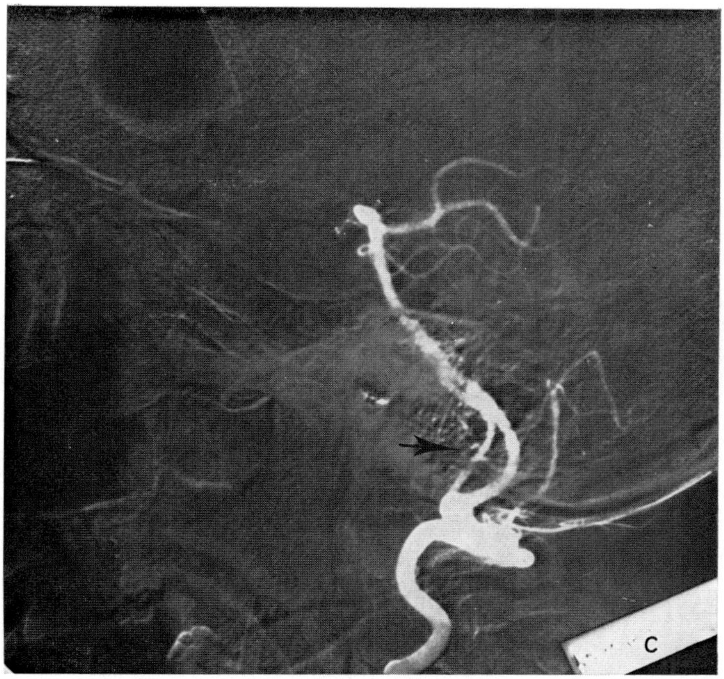

Fig. 1c

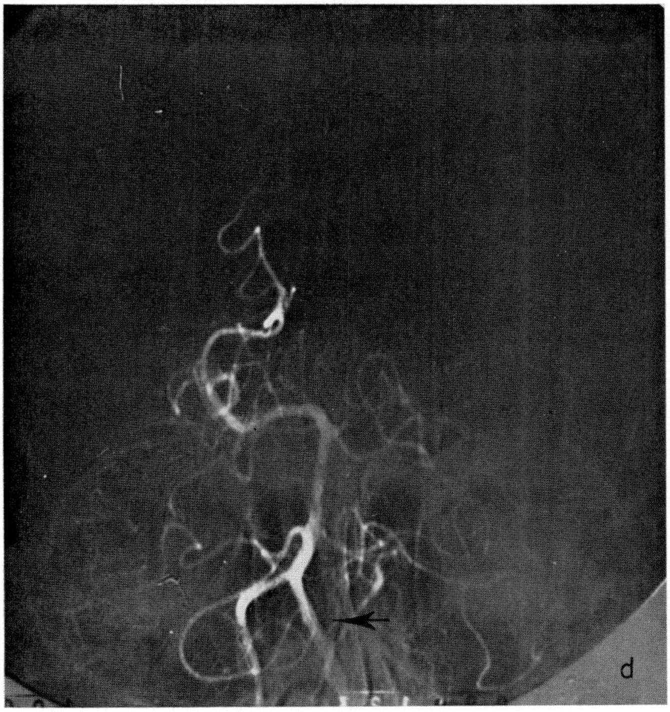

Fig. 1d

Fig. 1. Meningioma inserted on the lower part of the clivus and anterior margin of foramen magnum. a) Pneumoencephalography. b) Tumoral blush on the carotid arteriography. c) and d) Displacement of both vertebral arteries. The left one was cut to allow the total removal of the tumor

operating microscope), and the limitation of the lateral extent of the operative field, not much wider than the odontoid process. On the other hand, it offers an important advantage over other anterior approaches in that, in case of voluntary or accidental dural opening, closure will be easier and will not be accompanied by the risk of a cerebrospinal fluid leak into a septic cavity in the absence of a communication with the nasopharyngeal space.

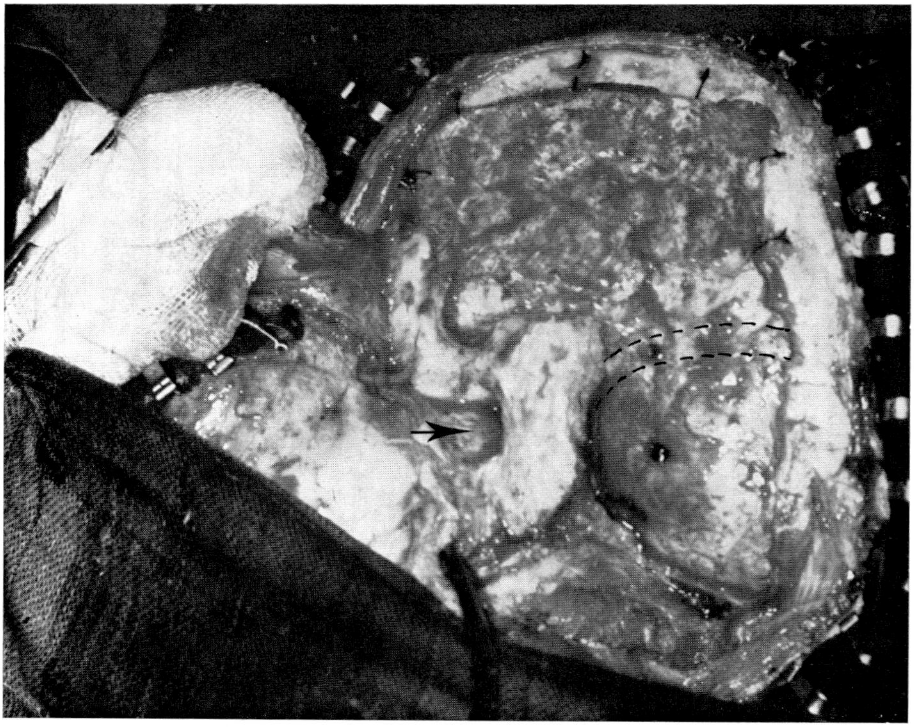

Fig. 2. Combination of a subtemporal and suboccipital approaches (extra dural view on a left side). The mastoid process is partially resected. The transverse sinus (dotted line) will be cut. Arrow = external auditory meatus

b) Transoral(-buccal) Approach

Just as the transcervical, the transoral approach also permits surgical exposure of the lower clival area. In our opinion, the latter is technically easier to perform. The patient is placed in a semisitting position with the head slightly rotated to the surgeon's side (a position similar to that used in transsphenoidal pituitary surgery). This position allows intraoperative fluoroscopy, permitting a better definition of the extent of bone removal and the visualization of the instrument tips. It also contributes to a rather dry surgical field by gravity drainage of all bleeding points. Care must be taken to pack the pharyngeal cavity with sponges to avoid pooling of blood and subsequent aspiration following extubation.

Many authors recommend preoperative tracheostomy. We do not consider it necessary. Tracheostomy can lead to postoperative complications such as infection of the pre-clival surgical field secondary to the accumulation of secretions often accompanying it. The endotracheal tube can be pushed to one side, out of the surgeon's field (Fig. 3). Tracheostomy is only indicated when postoperative oedema of the tongue is anticipated, an event that can be avoided by retracting the tongue mildly and which happens rarely when working above the C_2 level.

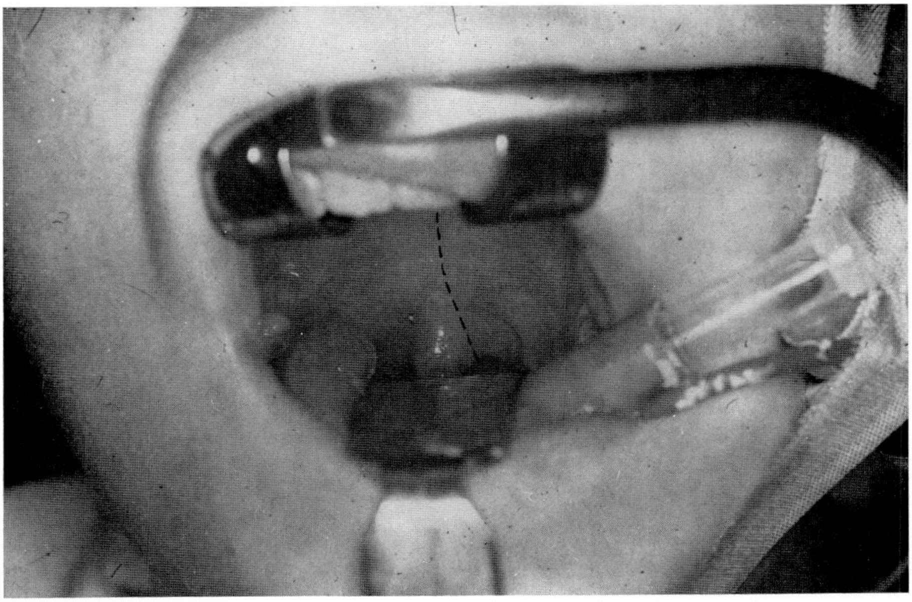

Fig. 3. Transoral approach. The endotracheal tube is pushed to one side, out of the surgeon's field. Notice the vertical incision of the soft palate (dotted line)

The operative field is widened by retraction of the soft palate. This can be accomplished by inserting two fine rubber catheters through the nares and brought out through the mouth. Often this is not sufficient, and the palate must be incised. We prefer a midline cut that extends from the hard palate to the uvula, where the incision becomes paramedian. Both sides of the soft palate are then retracted laterally as if they were a curtain. The incision may be extended by resecting the posterior edge of the bony palate, the so called transpalatal approach. The mucosa should be closed in two planes using absorbable material.

The anterior aspect of C_3, C_2, and C_1 is exposed by a midline vertical incision of the pharyngeal mucosa. The odontoid and the clivus can be seen after removal of the anterior arch of the Atlas. Extradural lesions such as chordomas and aneurysmal bone cysts can be easily removed using this route. Resection of the odontoid and the inferior clivus opens the anterior rim of the foramen magnum permitting extradural decompression of the brain stem in cases of cranio-vertebral junction anomalies or tumors of this region.

Tumoral invasion of the dura, on the other hand, is very difficult to attack transorally. This approach does not permit suture of the dura.

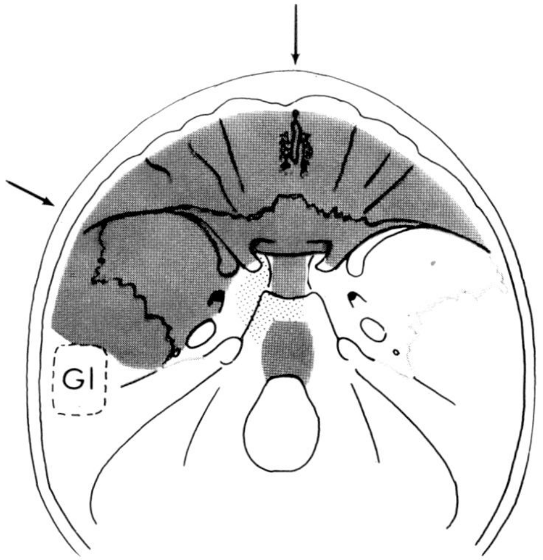

Fig. 4. Possibilities of exposure and resection of the base of the skull through an extradural and bifrontal approach

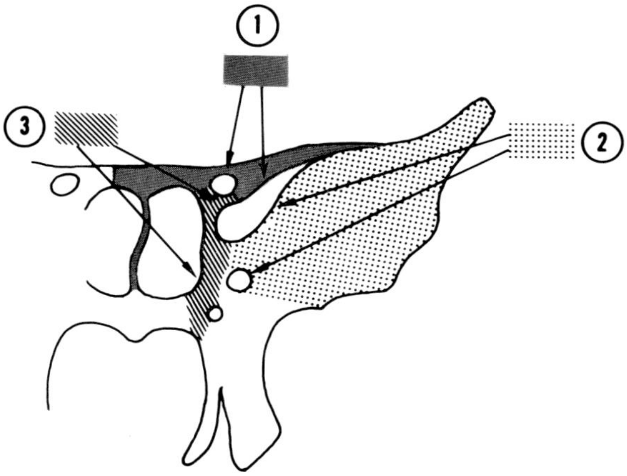

Fig. 5. Opening of the optic canal, sphenoid fissure, foramen rotundum and ovale after the resection of the sphenoid with: *1* a vertical attack, *2* a lateral attack, *3* a medial attack

Instead, one must resort to careful packing with muscle, aponeurosis, or lyophylized dura, risking a cerebrospinal fluid leak and meningitis. The latter is a danger in the use of this approach in the surgery of aneurysms of the lower third of the basilar artery. To be safe, the transoral approach should be reserved for the treatment of extradural lesions.

c) Transsphenoidal (rhino-septal) Approach

This well known technique is extensively used in pituitary surgery. It is also the most simple approach to obtain tissue biopsy of deeply seated tumors, as well as for the removal of soft neoplasms limited to the sphenoid

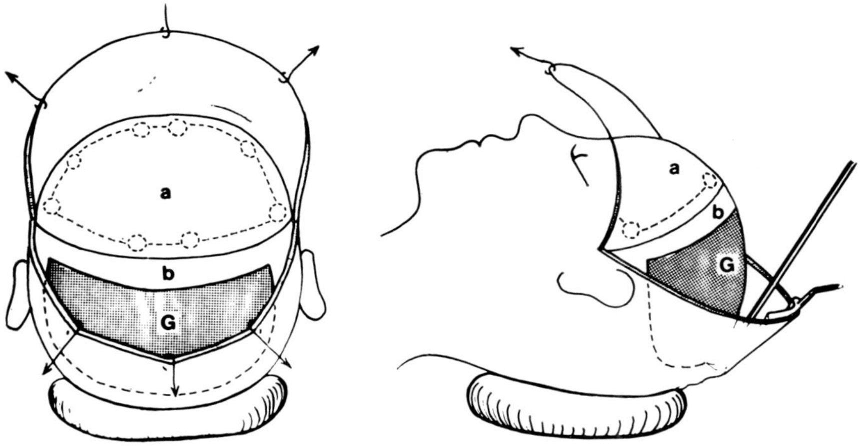

Fig. 6. Extracting a pericranial graft on the biparietal area. *a* anterior pericranium, *G* graft, *b* pericranial band preserved to allow a suture at the end of the procedure

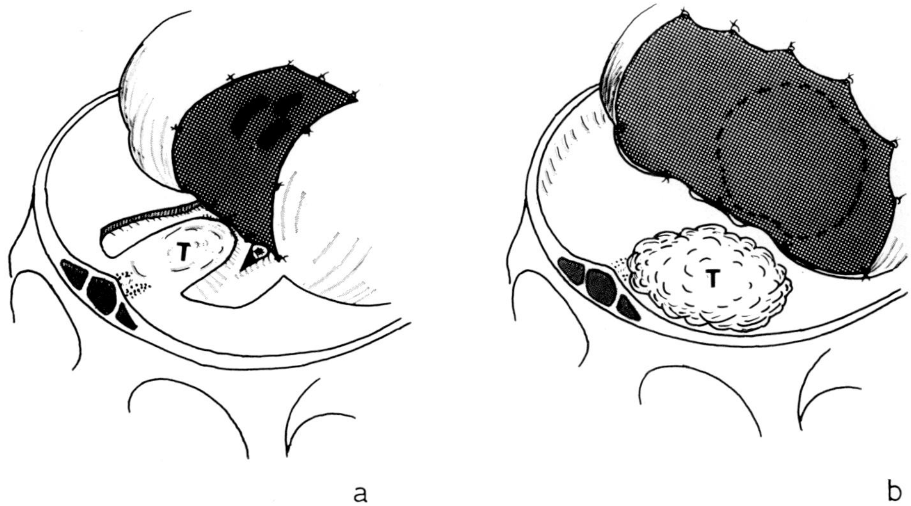

Fig. 7. Repair of the dura. a) Suture of meningeal tears and strenghtening on the midline with a pericranial graft. b) Dural defect closed with a large graft sutured at the posterior edges of the anterior fossa. *T* tumor

sinus. The upper half of the clivus can also be reached, but its approach is limited by the interposition of the sella turcica, and it is facilitated by an ample sphenoid sinus, especially a large posterior recess with a thin clival wall.

The rhino-septal route permits excellent visualization of midline structures, but it provides a narrow, 10 to 12 mm, surgical window, through which one cannot remove a hard tumor, nor a tumor that extends to the body of the sphenoid. The optic nerves, of course, cannot be visualized either.

Whereas rhinorrhea secondary to pituitary surgery is rather easy to control by local measures, it is much more difficult to control when it

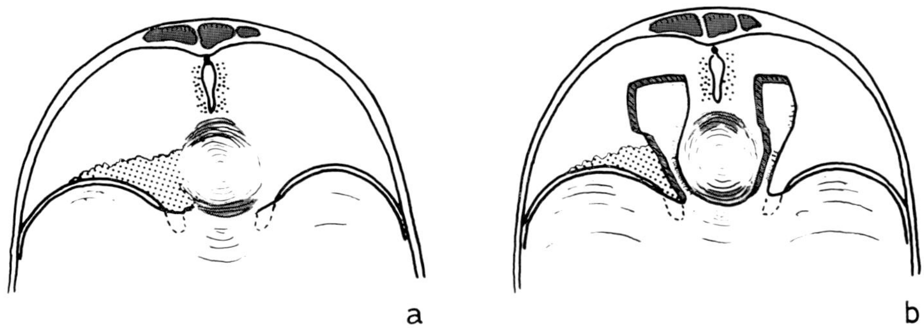

Fig. 8. a) Fibrous dysplasia involving the sphenoidal body and the left lesser wing. b) Exposing the extra dural portion of the optic nerves

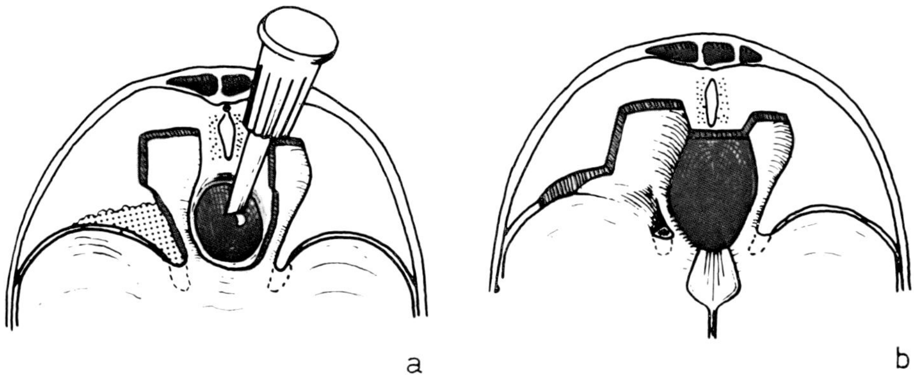

Fig. 9. a) Intra tumoral resection between the optic nerves. b) The total removal of the sphenoid body leads to the pharyngeal mucosae and nasal fossae. Opening of the left sphenoid fissure and resection of the left anterior clinoid process

occurs during extrasellar, transsphenoidal surgery, necessitating careful packing of the sphenoid sinus with muscle and bone grafts. Because of the danger of secondary meningeal infection, this approach is also preferred in cases of extradural pathology.

d) Transbasal Approach

This approach is a modification of the surgical techniques developed by Tessier *et al.*[14] in the treatment of cranio-facial malformations. After a bicoronal, bifrontal opening, the dura is dissected away from the base of the

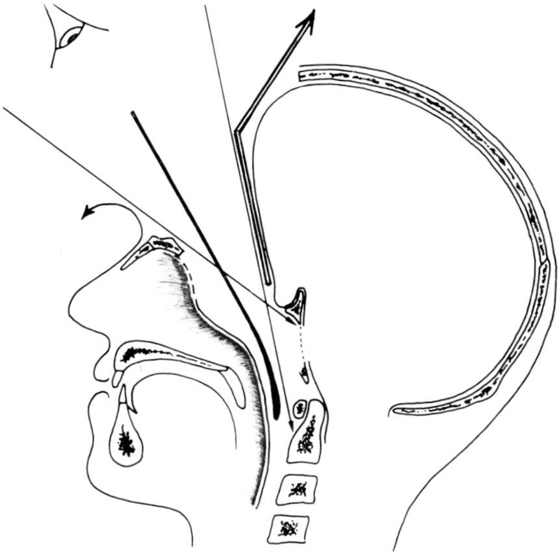

Fig. 10. After the resection of the sphenoid body it is possible to reach the anterior rim of foramen magnum, C_1 and C_2, preserving the pharyngeal mucosae

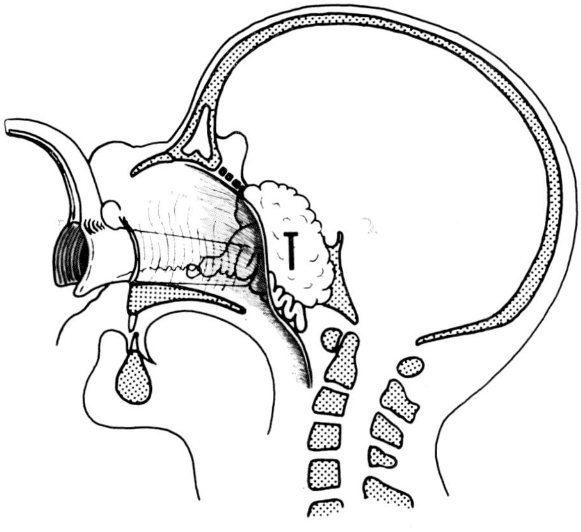

Fig. 11. Through a rhino-septal approach the rhinopharyngeal mucosae can be preserved. Packing is introduced both for protection and deep landmarks

skull; the olfactory nerves must be cut at the level of the cribiform plate. The plane can be carried as far back as the petrous bones, exposing the anterior and middle fossae (Fig. 4). With careful technique it is possible to dissect cleanly the neurovascular structures that pass through the optic canal, the sphenoid fissure, the foramen rotundum, and foramen ovale, freeing them from any tumor (Fig. 5).

This procedure removes most of the tissue interphase between the subarachnoid space and nasopharynx, making imperative the strict application of certain principles to avoid complications. Any dural tears must be

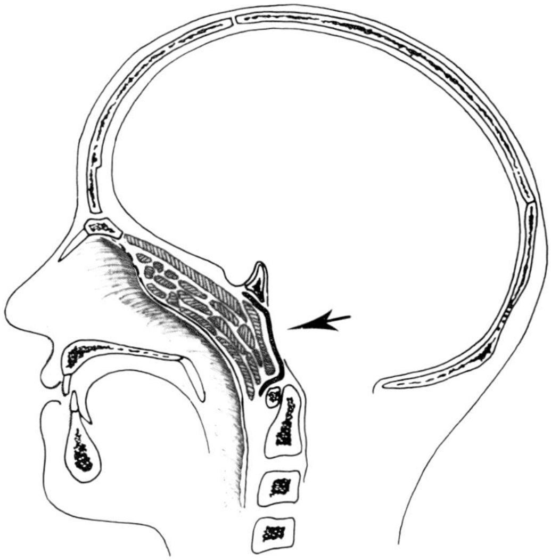

Fig. 12. Repair of a clival dural defect with a pericranial graft applied by bone reconstruction

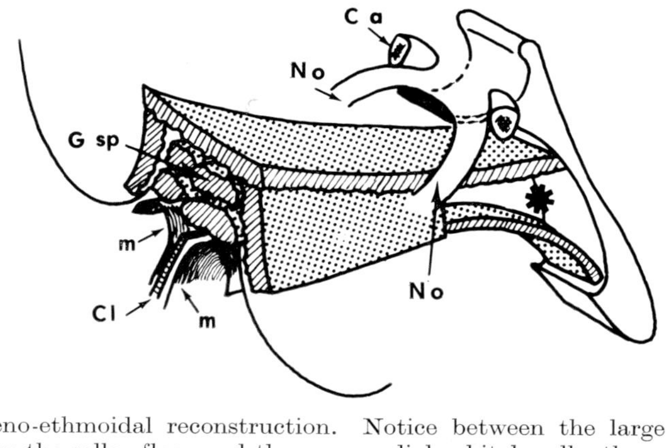

Fig. 13. Spheno-ethmoidal reconstruction. Notice between the large upper graft impacted below the sellar floor and the new medial orbital walls, the packing of the dead space with cancellous bone grafts (*G sp*). Both optic nerves are free (*No*). *Ca* tip of anterior clinoid process, *m* mucosae, *Cl* nasal septum

tightly closed and reinforced with pericranium, thus avoiding a cerebrospinal fluid leak and an ascending infection (Fig. 6). The base of the skull must be reconstructed with bone autografts, eliminating any dead space that might encourage extradural hematomas, abscesses, or meningoencephaloceles. The nasopharyngeal mucosal plane must be preserved, for

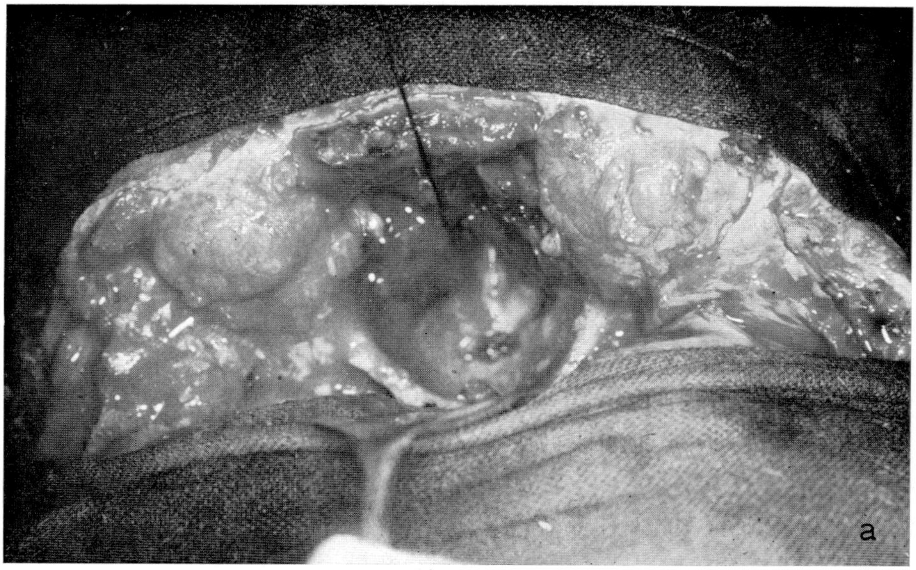

Fig. 14a

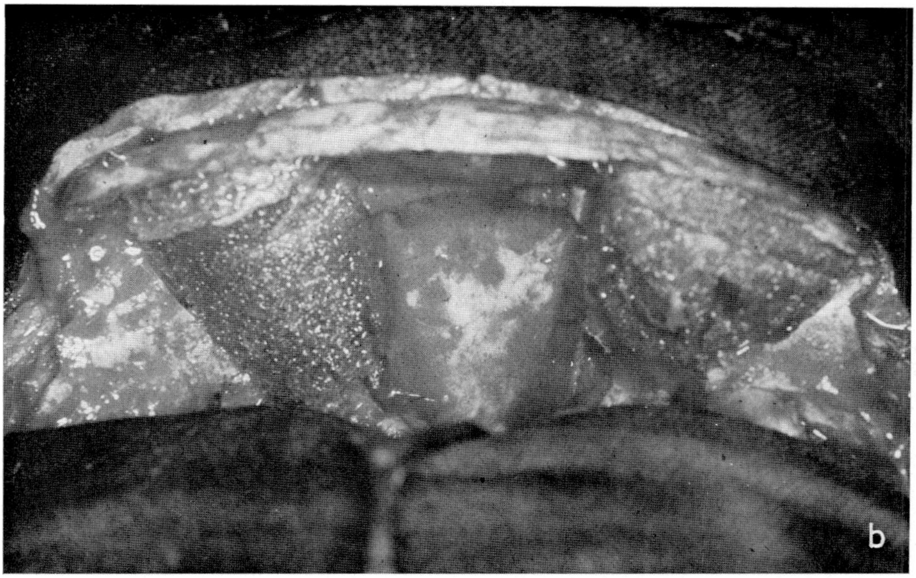

Fig. 14b

Fig. 14. Fibrous dysplasia at the base of the skull. a) Resection of the whole anterior fossa. Between the optic nerves and the sphenoid fissures one reaches the pharyngeal mucosa. b) Repair of the spheno-ethmoidal area and orbital roofs with iliac autografts. Reconstruction of the supra orbital margins with a modelled split rib graft

it provides physical support as well as vascularization to the bone grafts. When these dicta are followed, the transbasal approach is rendered a benign procedure.

The following are some guidelines and technical notes for the surgery of tumors of the sphenoid and clivus:

I. Bicoronal incision.
II. Low bifrontal free-bone flap, if necessary passing through the frontal sinuses.
III. Dissection of the subfrontal dura to the posterior limits of the anterior fossa.
IV. Suture repair of any meningeal tear and reinforcement with pericranium graft (Figs. 7 a and b).

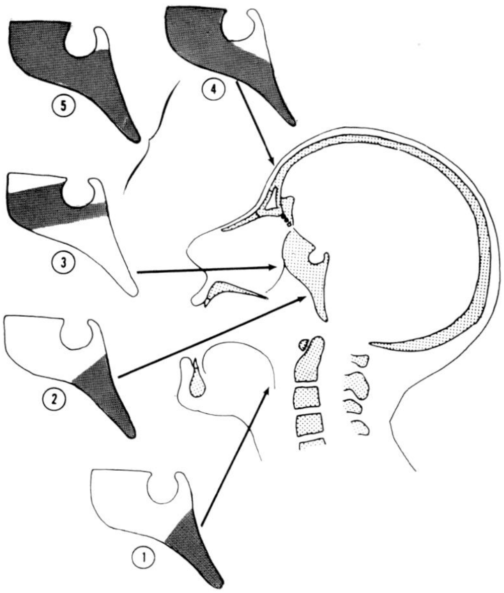

Fig. 15. Limits of sphenoidal and clival resection through anterior approaches. *1* Transcervical, *2* transoral, *3* transphenoidal, *4* transbasal, *5* transbasal and rhinoseptal in combination

V. Partial resection of the posterior orbital roof and optic canal, exposing the extradural portion of the optic nerves (Figs. 8 a and b).
VI. Midline attack of the tumor between the optic nerves, through the planum sphenoidale (Fig. 9 a).
VII. In the case of lateral extension of the tumor, resection of the lesser and greater wings of the sphenoid, opening of the orbital fissure and the foramina rotundum and ovale, if necessary.
VIII. Intratumoral resection.
IX. Combined lateral and midline resection of tumor and bony margins leading to the total removal of the sphenoid body in front of the sellar floor (Figs. 9 a and b).
X. Exposure of the submucosal nasopharyngeal plane along the extracranial portion of the clivus to the anterior rim of the foramen

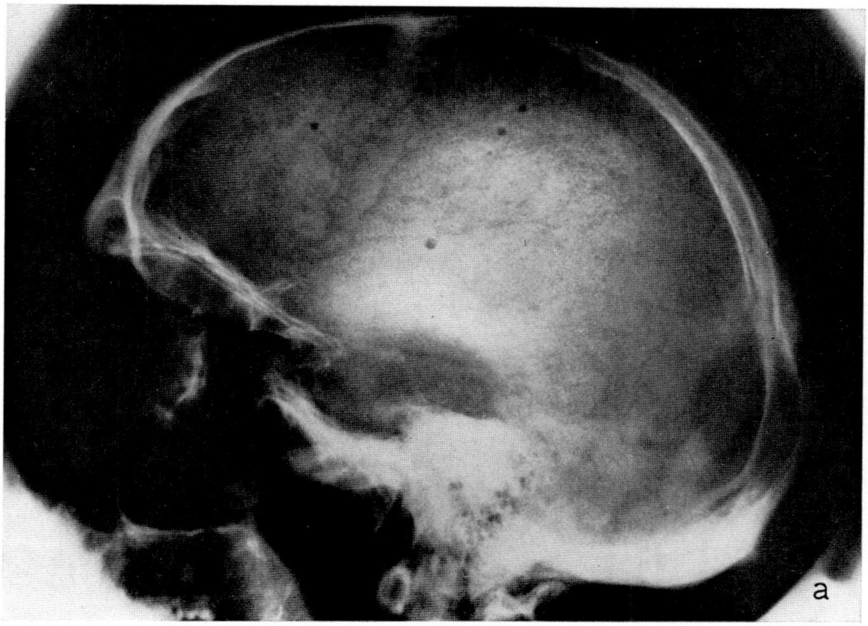

Fig. 16a

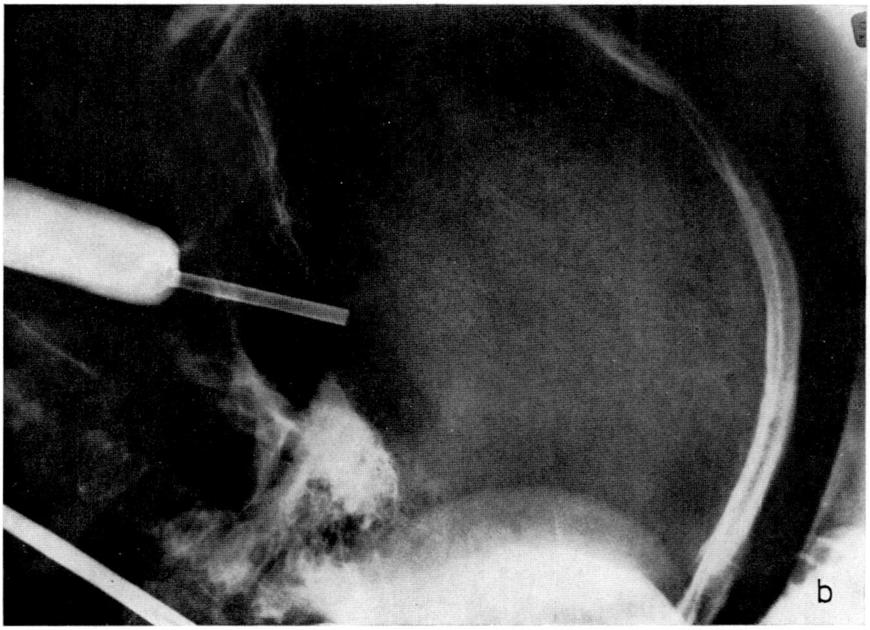

Fig. 16b

Fig. 16. A rhino-septal biopsy is necessary. a) Radiological aspect of sphenoidal tumor with clival and sellar destruction. b) Pre-operative biopsy; sphenoidal mucocele. Air is filling the empty cavity and the tip of the instrument is on the clival dura

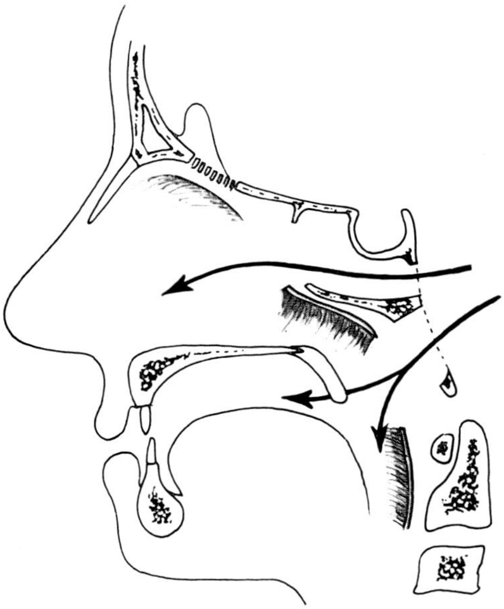

Fig. 17. The risk of post-operative CSF leakage is higher in the case of transoral or rhino-septal approaches because these are transmucosal routes

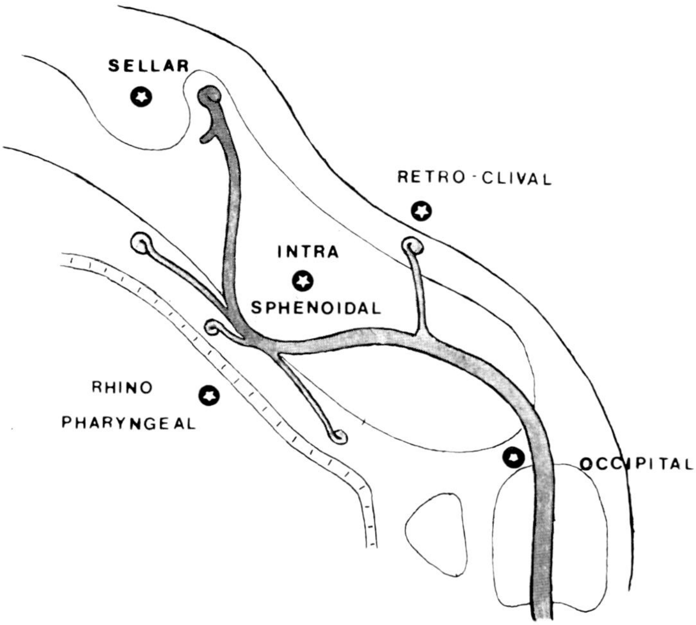

Fig. 18. The various sites of clival chordomas are the results of the multiple expansions of the notochord

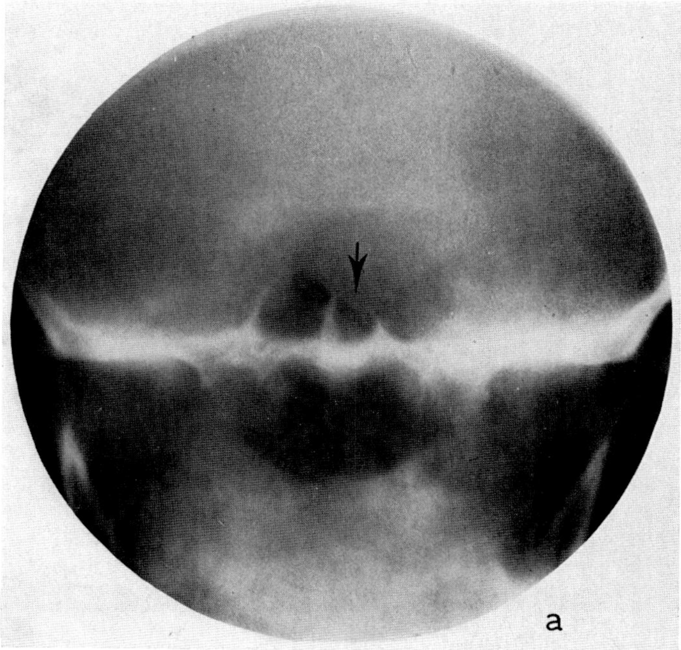

Fig. 19a

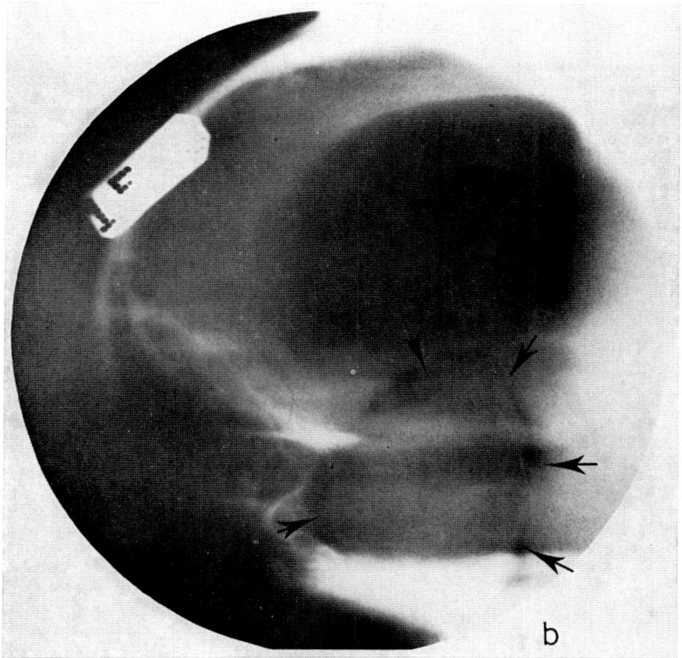

Fig. 19b

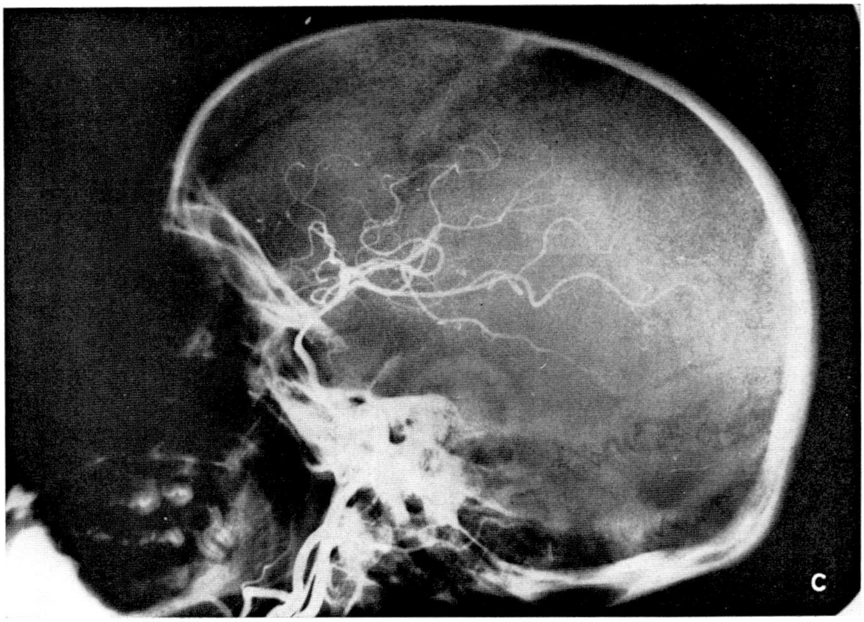

Fig. 19c

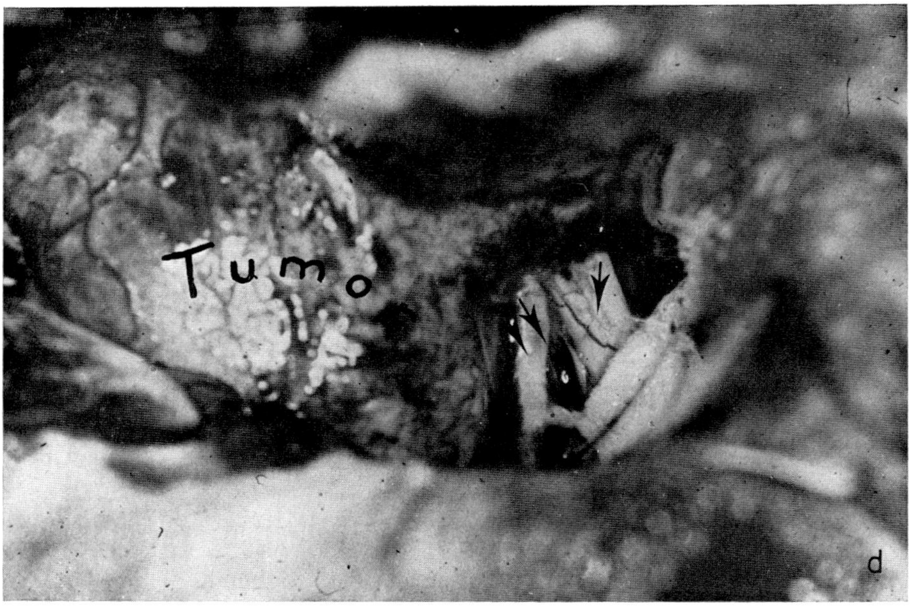

Fig. 19d

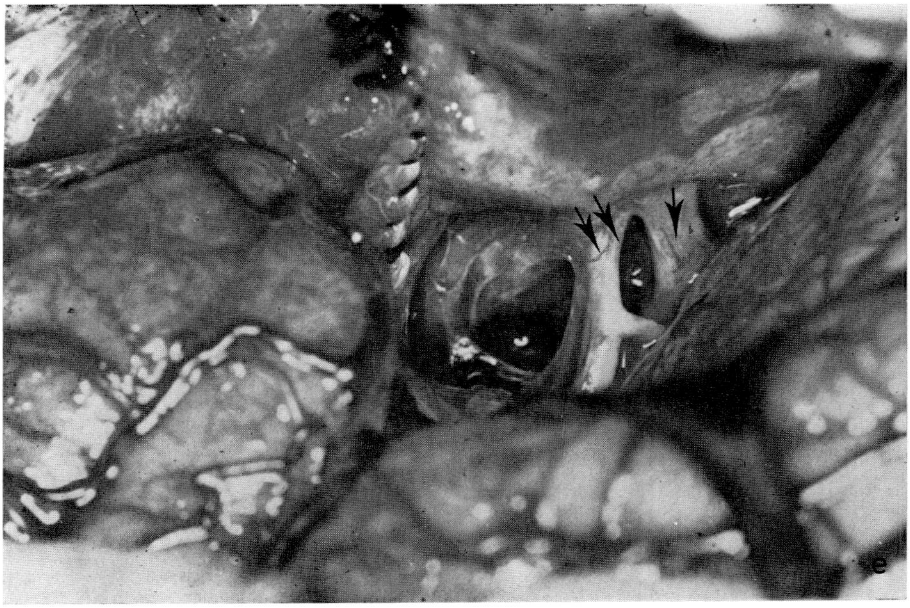

Fig. 19e

Fig. 19. Intradural approach in a case of chordoma involving the cavernous sinus. a) "Double Floor" of the sella. b) Pneumoencephalography (parasagittal cut). c) Stretching of the left carotid artery. d) Bulging of the tumor in the cavernous sinus and temporal areas, still covered with the dura. e) After the removal of the tumor, the dural incision is sutured and left optic nerve (single arrow) and left carotid artery (double arrow) decompressed

magnum and the anterior border of C_1, C_2, and C_3, if necessary (Fig. 10).

XI. When necessary, the rhino-septal approach can be used to develop the rhinopharyngeal mucosal plane. This procedure should immediately precede the transbasal opening (Fig. 11).

XII. Removal of the sellar floor.

XIII. Removal of the clivus until healthy bone or dura is reached.

XIV. Repair of any clival dural defects with pericranium (Fig. 12).

XV. Extraction of iliac bone grafts (cancellous bone is better than cortical bone as donor).

XVI. Reconstruction of the sphenoid mass, medial orbital walls and orbital roofs. Optic nerves must remain completely free (Figs. 13, 14 a and b).

XVII. Closure.

In spite of the expected postoperative anosmia and the rather lengthy surgical session (about 10 hours), this procedure is remarkably well tolerated by the patient, as with other extradural procedures. Postoperative risks of cerebrospinal fluid leak and meningitis secondary to tears of the clival dura are minimized because of the submucosal nature of the approach.

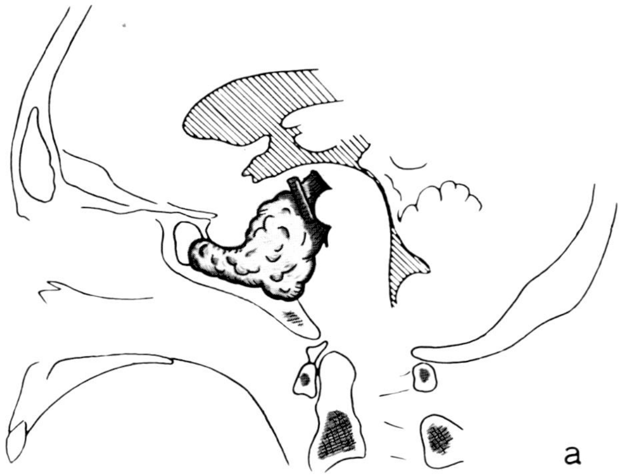

Fig. 20a

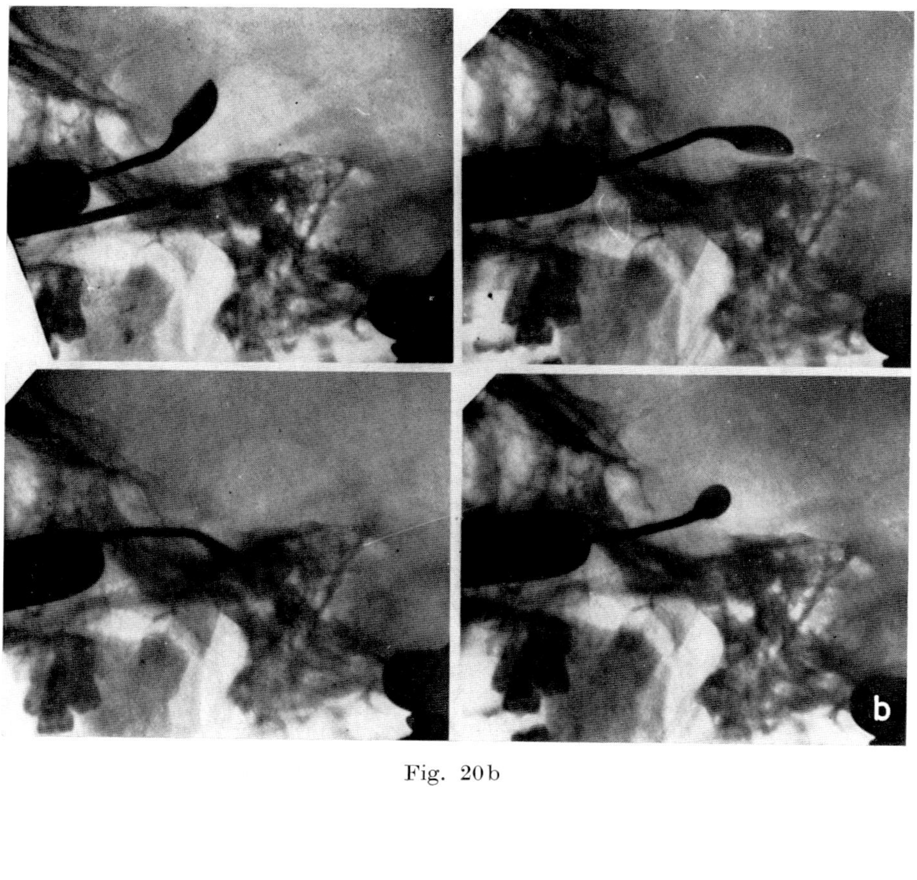

Fig. 20b

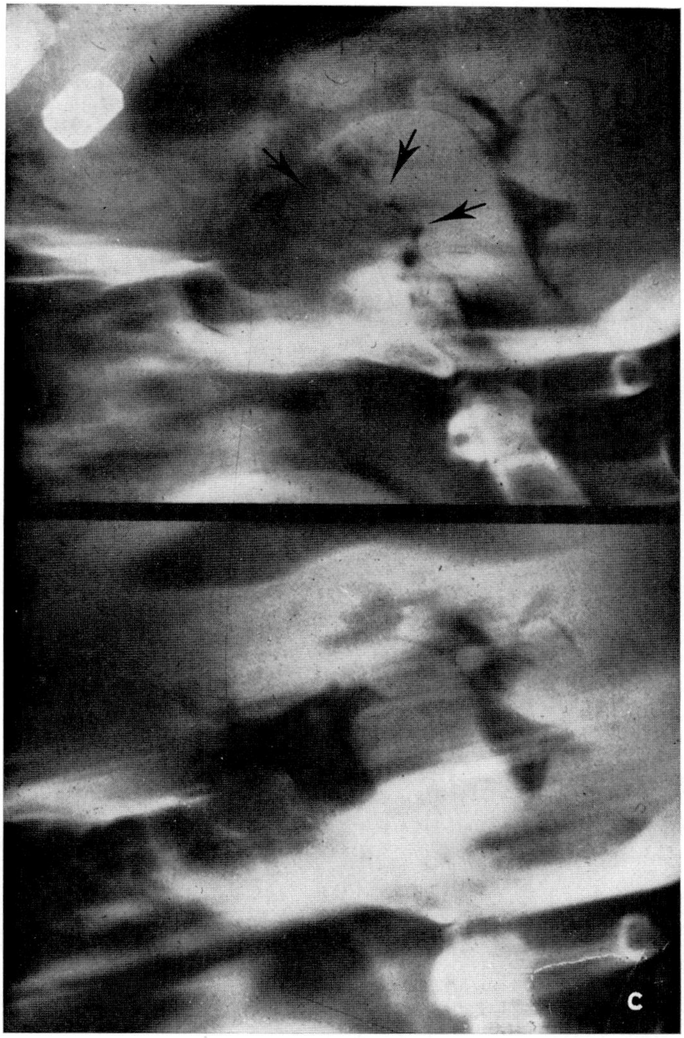

Fig. 20c

Fig. 20. Chordoma approached by the rhino-septal route. a) The tumor involves the sphenoidal sinus and the upper half of the clivus. b) Positions of the instruments during the transphenoidal removal. c) Comparison between pre- and post-operative pneumo-encephalography

In summary (Fig. 15), the transcervical and transoral approaches permit access to the lower half of the clivus; the transphenoidal route allows exposure of the upper half of the clivus strictly on the midline. The transbasal procedure is the only approach that permits surgical exposure and removal of tumors extending from the floor of the anterior fossa as far caudal as the level of C_2. Only the clival area, sheltered by the sella cannot be reached transbasally. However, this area can be reached transphenoidally,

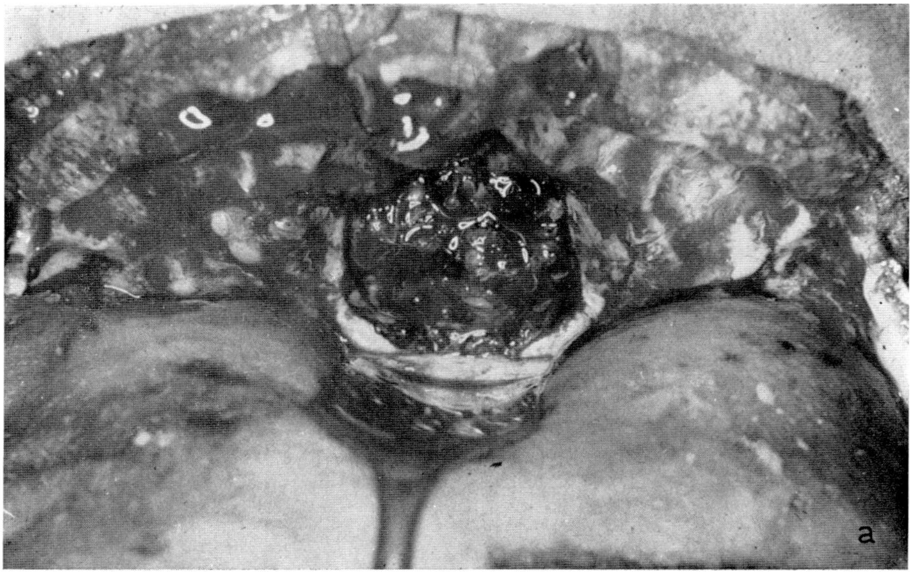

Fig. 21a

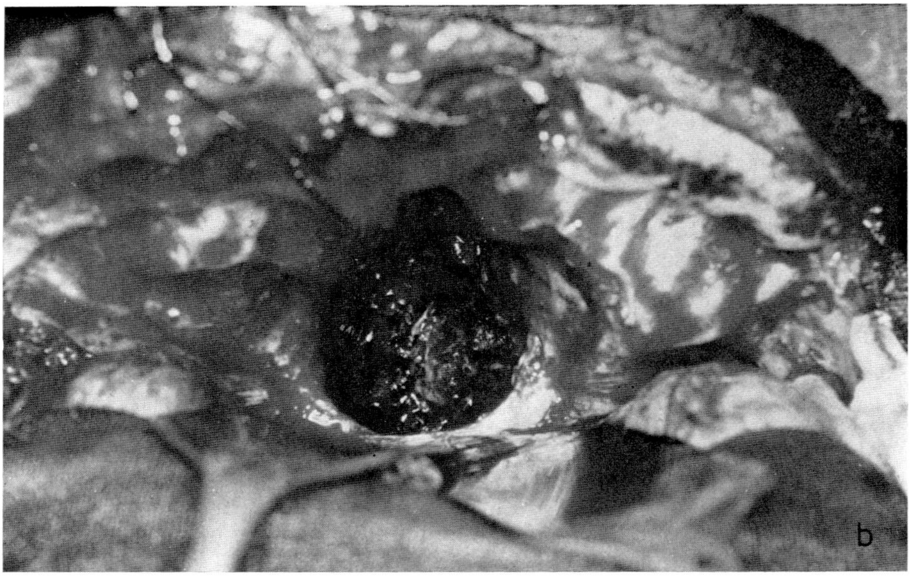

Fig. 21b

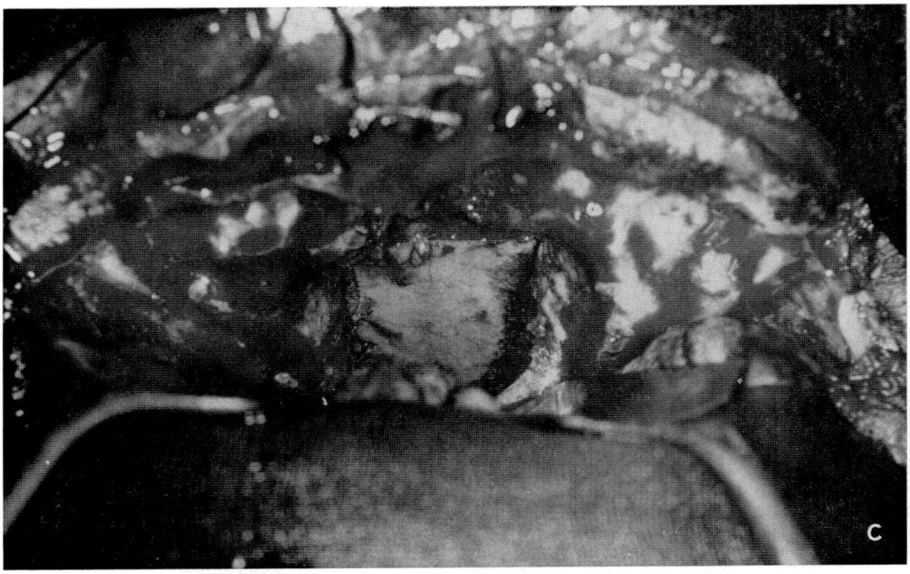

Fig. 21c

Fig. 21. Transbasal approach in a case of spheno-ethmoidal chordoma. a) The extradural compression of both optic nerves is responsible for visual disturbancies. b) After the removal, notice the pharyngeal mucosa between the free optic nerves. c) Reconstruction of the spheno-ethmoidal area. Notice the large upper graft

and we often combine the two approaches as is deemed necessary. The transphenoidal approach to the clivus is facilitated by the resection of sphenoid bone accomplished transbasally. Only the dorsum sellae and the posterior clinoids cannot be reached by these combined procedures, necessitating for their removal an intradural approach.

III. Choice of Surgical Approach

1. Biopsy

When the usual battery of tests does not help the surgeon in establishing a preoperative diagnosis and in choosing a surgical approach, a biopsy of a sphenoidal tumor becomes necessary. The biopsy is usually obtained transphenoidally. It provides the surgeon with a histological diagnosis, and in addition it gives information as to the consistency of the tumor. Frequently, patients presumed to have a large, inoperable chordoma, have instead a benign sphenoidal mucocele. The clinical history and symptomatology of these two entities is often quite similar, *i.e.*, headaches, transitory oculomotor palsies, occasional visual disturbances, with a radiological picture of destruction of the sphenoid body and erosion of the bony edges of the sphenoid sinus and sellar floor. Transphenoidal biopsy in these cases, not only provides the diagnosis but may also cure the patient (Figs. 16 a and b).

2. *Tumor Relation to the Dura*

It is important to emphasize that among the various techniques described above, some respect the mucosal plane and some do not. When the mucosa

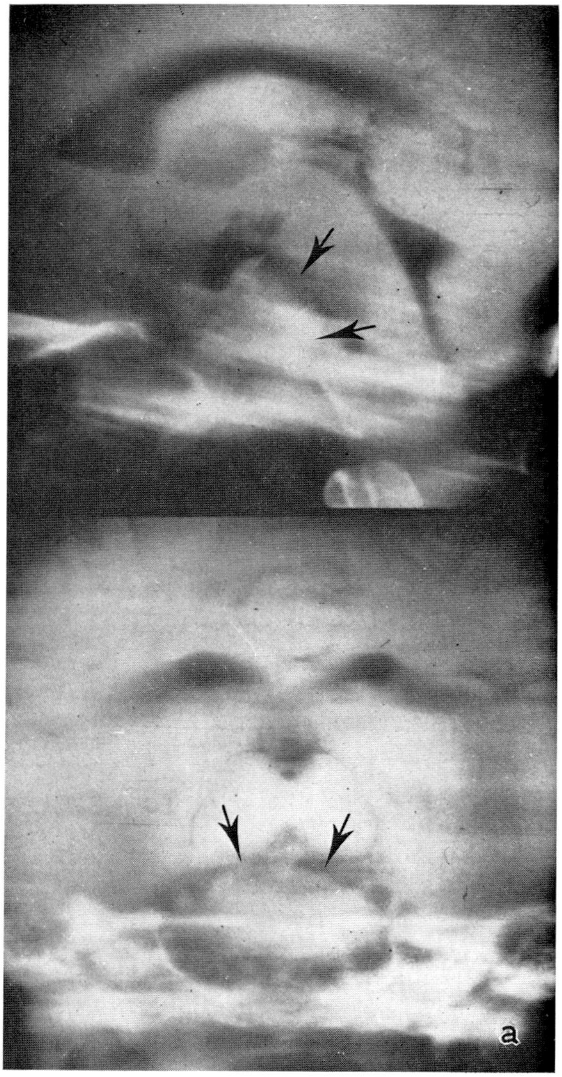

Fig. 22a

is opened, as in the transphenoidal and transoral approaches, the postoperative risk of meningitis becomes real following a tear in the clival dura. Closure of the dural defect is more hazardous in the transoral approach, where the mere suture of the pharyngeal mucosa is usually insufficient to prevent cerebrospinal fluid leakage. The transbasal approach, on the other

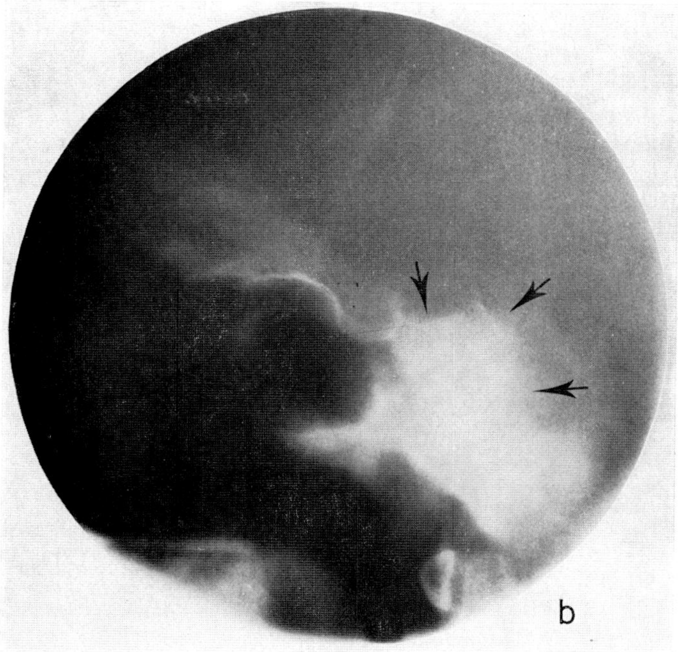

Fig. 22b

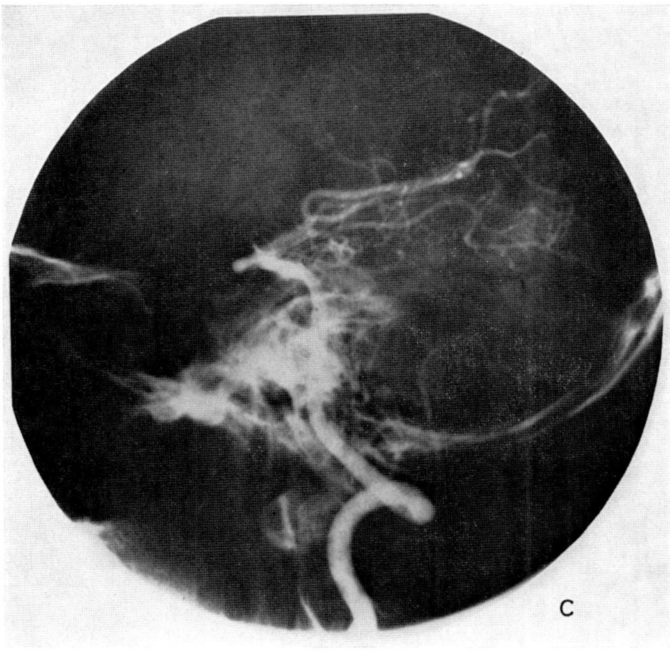

Fig. 22c

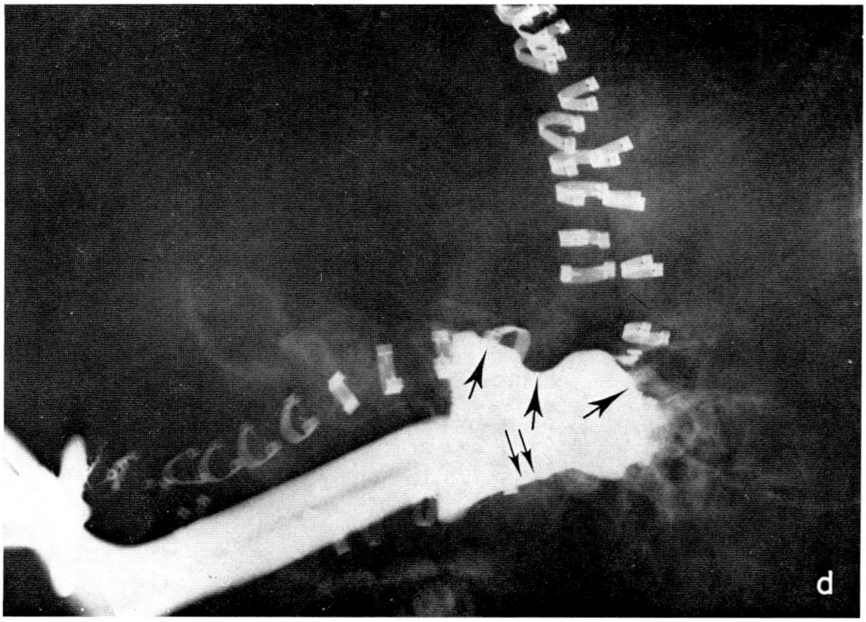

Fig. 22d

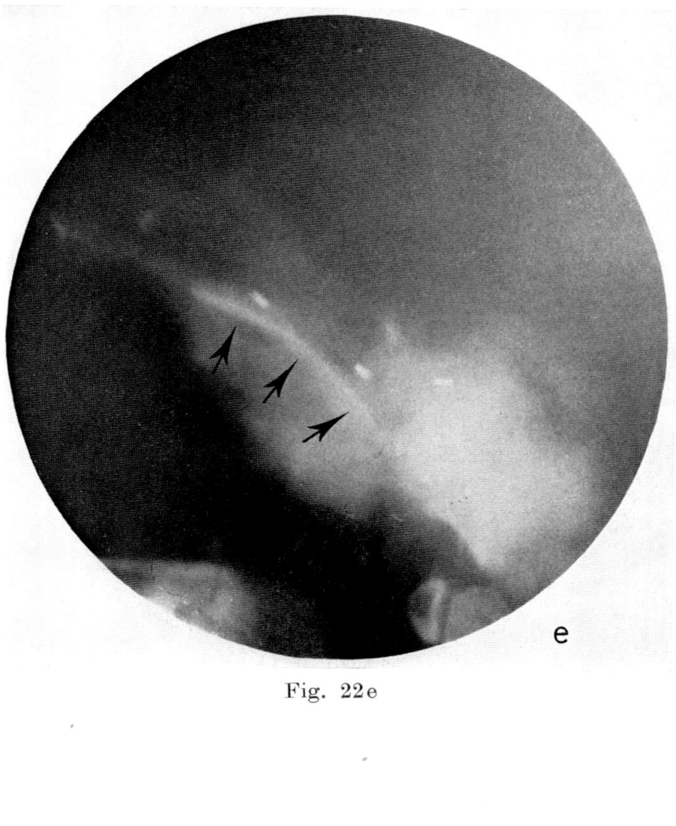

Fig. 22e

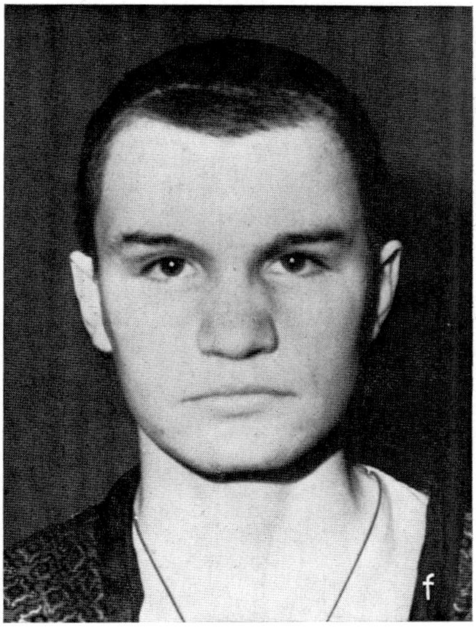

Fig. 22f

Fig. 22. First case of combined rhino-septal and transbasal approaches in one stage. a) Incomplete removal of the chordoma after a first rhino-septal procedure (post-operative pneumoencephalography). b) Calcified recurrence two years later. c) Distorsion of the basilar artery explaining drop attacks. d) Combined approaches. Intra-operative radiography with pantopaque filling the empty cavity after the tumor removal. The arrows show the subfrontal, sellar and clival dura. The mucosa (double arrow) is preserved. e) Post-operative tomography of the reconstruction. Clips are on the subfrontal, sellar and clival dura. Notice the large upper graft (arrows). f) The patient one month after the procedure

hand, minimizes cerebrospinal fluid leakages and meningitis by preserving the integrity of the mucosal plane, by making it possible to repair meningeal tears, and by permitting bony reconstruction, assuring a tighter closure. Moreover, when tumor spread necessitates an intradural approach, the latter can be combined with the transbasal procedure.

Thus, the choice of approach, depends in part on the position of the tumor with respect to the dura. A pure intradural tumor such as a clival meningioma, should not be approached anteriorly. When an extradural neoplasm invades the dura, the "submucosal", rather than the "trans-mucosal" route is recommended (Fig. 17).

3. *Consistency of the Tumor*

The consistency of the tumor also dictates what procedure to follow. Hard tumors are removed with the help of rongeurs, drills and chisels. These tumors often exert extradural compression on the upper cranial nerves. Their surgical decompression dictates the transbasal approach.

On the other hand, soft tumors that can be removed with spoons and suction can be attacked via a narrow surgical field such as that offered by transphenoidal surgery, often irrespective of their size.

4. Histology

The choice of surgery also depends on the histology of the lesion (usually obtained via a transphenoidal approach). One should attempt total removal of an extensive, benign tumor. It is wrong to propose an extensive procedure in case of a malignant tumor, when total removal is deemed impossible, as for example, when the cavernous sinus is involved. In these cases, the more benign transphenoidal procedure followed by radiotherapy is prefered.

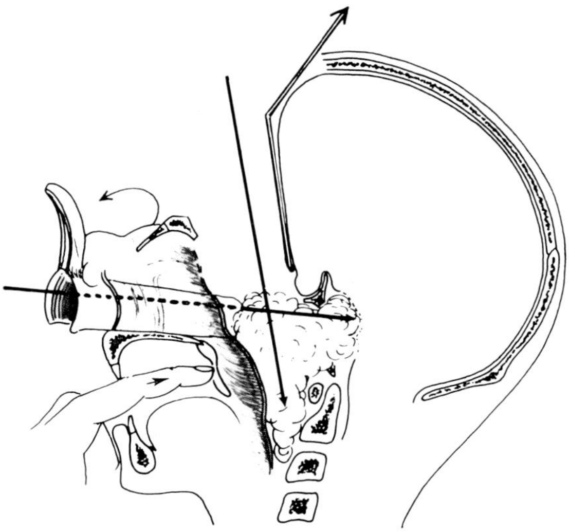

Fig. 23. Combination of several approaches during the same procedure (transbasal, rhino-septal and "pseudotransoral" routes)

5. Localization and Extent of the Tumor

The choice of the approach is in great part determined by the location of the tumor as well as by its extent. This point is best illustrated in the case of chordomas, histologically benign tumors of the midline sphenoidal-clival region. They can grow and extend in any direction, and may invade the dura, becoming also intradural neoplasms (Fig. 18). Their surgical treatment is best determined by considering all the parameters previously mentioned. The most complete removal possible, followed by radiotherapy affords long survival and perhaps cure.

a) Intradural Approach

This type of approach can be used when the tumor appears purely intradural, without obvious bone invasion, as is the case with meningiomas of the clival area. It can be used also in cases where the tumor invades structures impossible to reach via an extradural route, as is the case with tumors near the cavernous sinus (Figs. 19 a, b, c, d, and e).

b) Extradural Approach

This is the most logical approach in case of an extradural tumor. Parenthetically, one should note that in the early stages, chordomas are purely extradural, making early diagnosis and treatment most desirable.

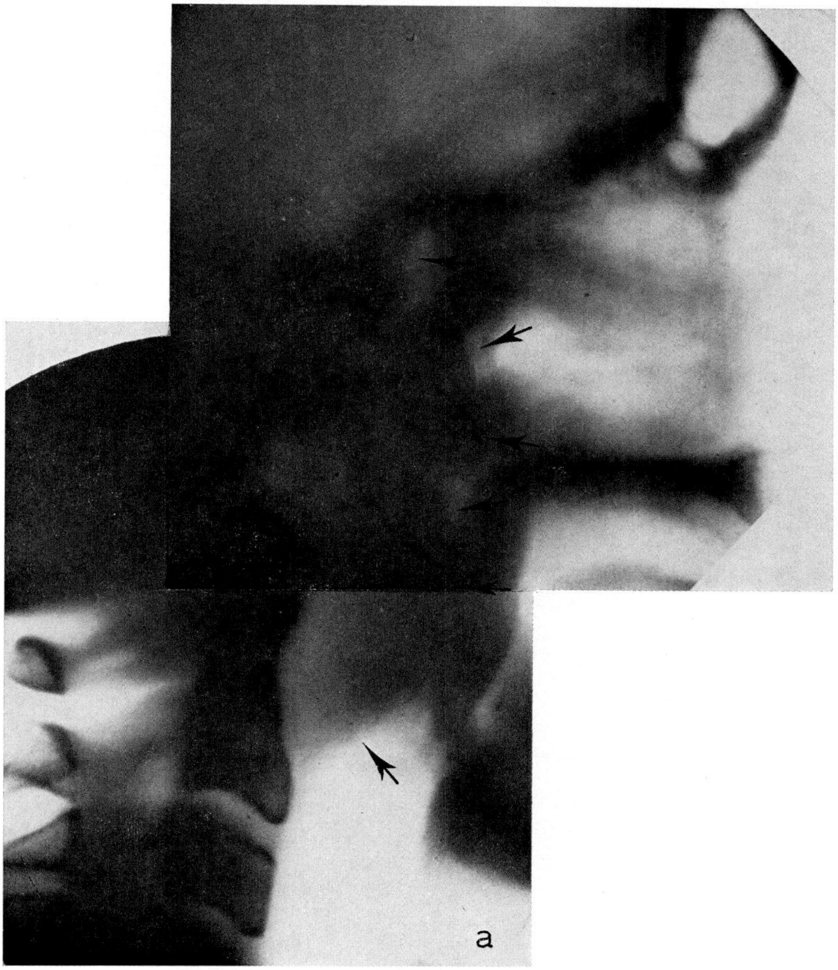

Fig. 24a

Transoral and cervical approaches can be used in tumors strictly limited to the lower half of the clivus. The transphenoidal route can be used in cases of soft tumors of the upper half of the clivus extending to the sphenoidal sinus (Figs. 20 a, b, and c). The transbasal approach is necessary when the body of the sphenoid is invaded (Figs. 21 a, b, and c), when there is

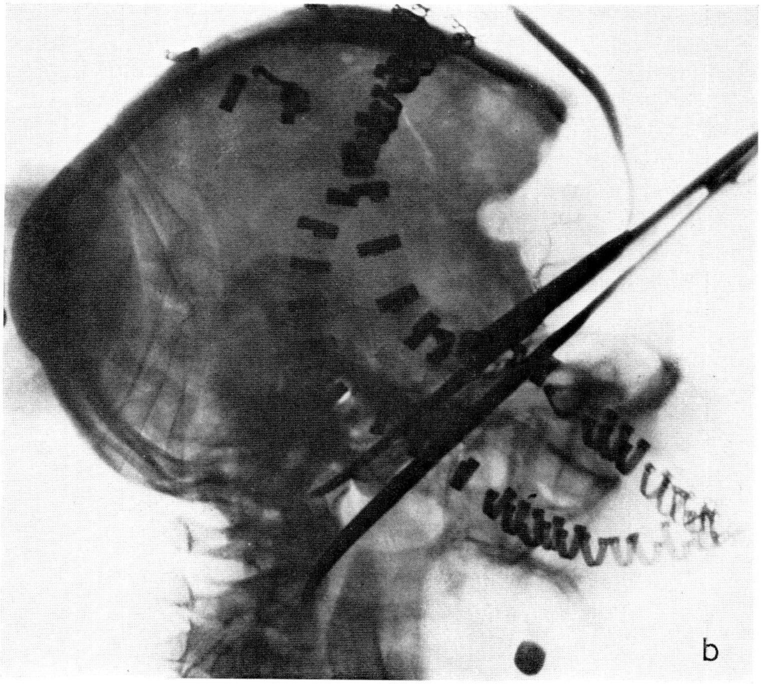

Fig. 24b

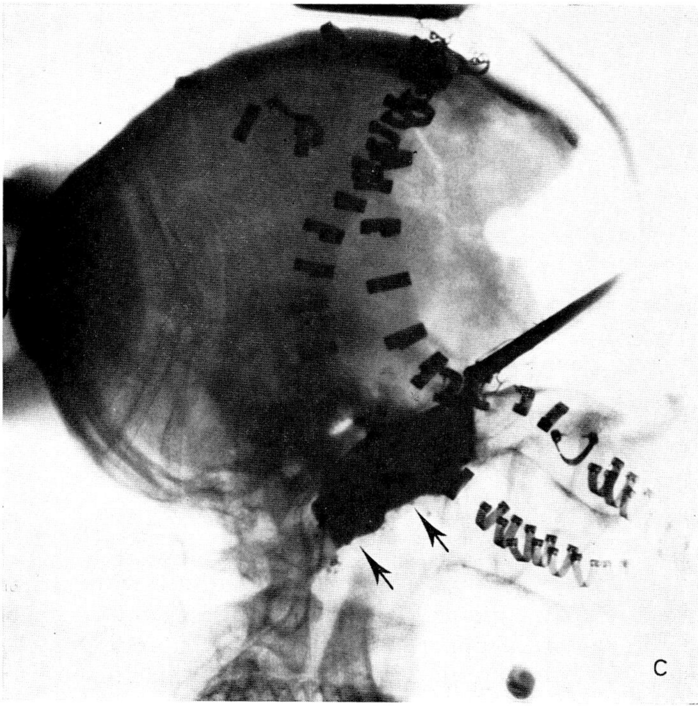

Fig. 24c

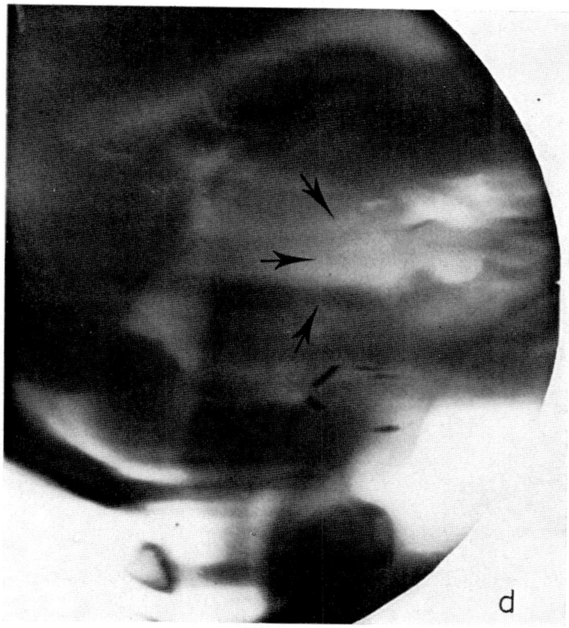

Fig. 24d

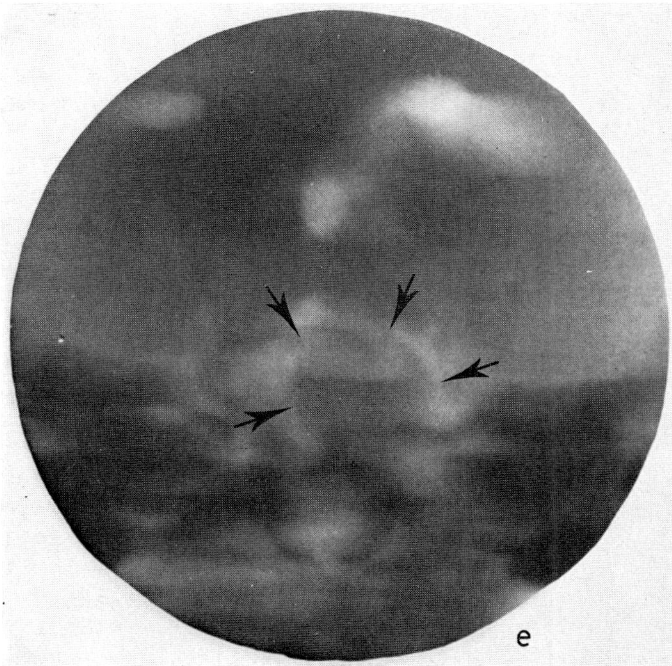

Fig. 24e

Fig. 24. Association of transbasal and intra-dural approaches in two stages. a) Preoperative tomography. The chordoma invades the sphenoidal sinus, obstructs the choanae and extends behind the soft palate. b) Intra-operative radiography during the transbasal procedure. The instrument tips are in front of foramen magnum and C_2. c) Intra-operative view where the empty cavity is filled with pantopaque after the removal of the tumor from the sphenoidal sinus to C_2. The pharyngeal mucosa (arrows) is preserved. d and e) Post-operative pneumoencephalography where the large graft repairing the base is visible. An interpeduncular expansion remains and was removed through a subtemporal approach 3 months after the first procedure

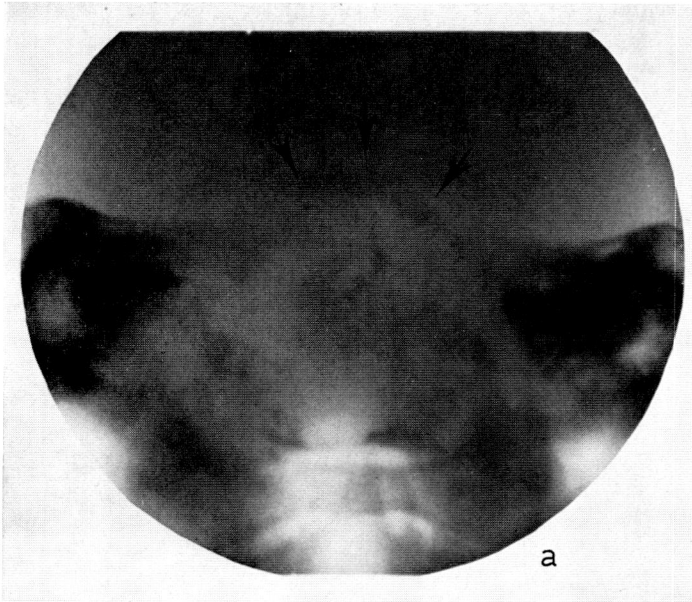

Fig. 25a

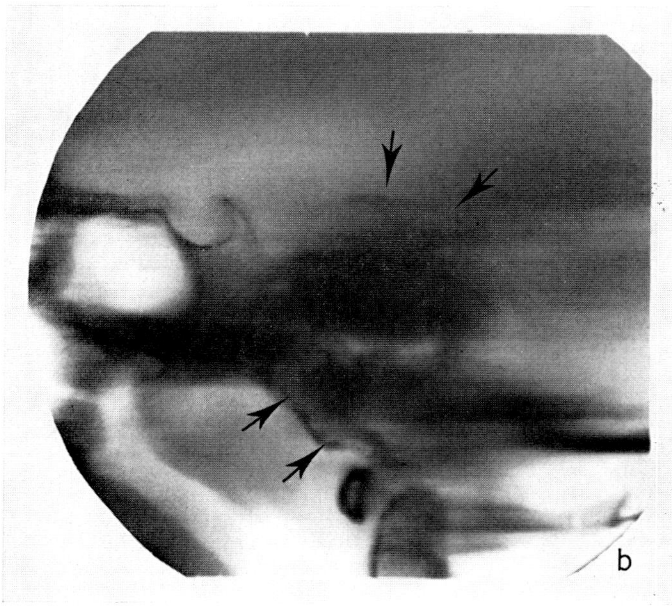

Fig. 25b

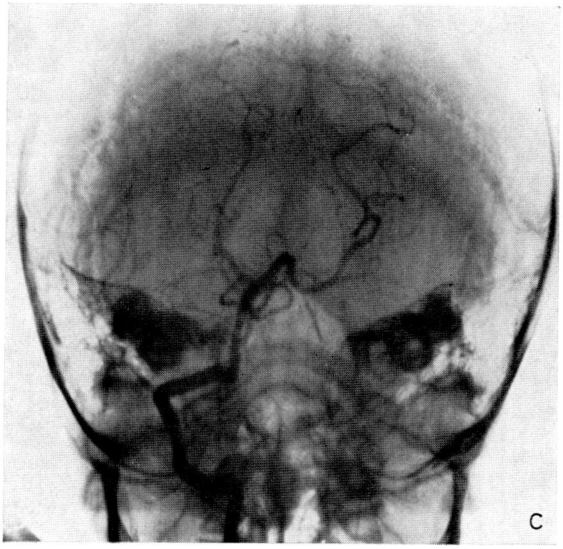

Fig. 25c

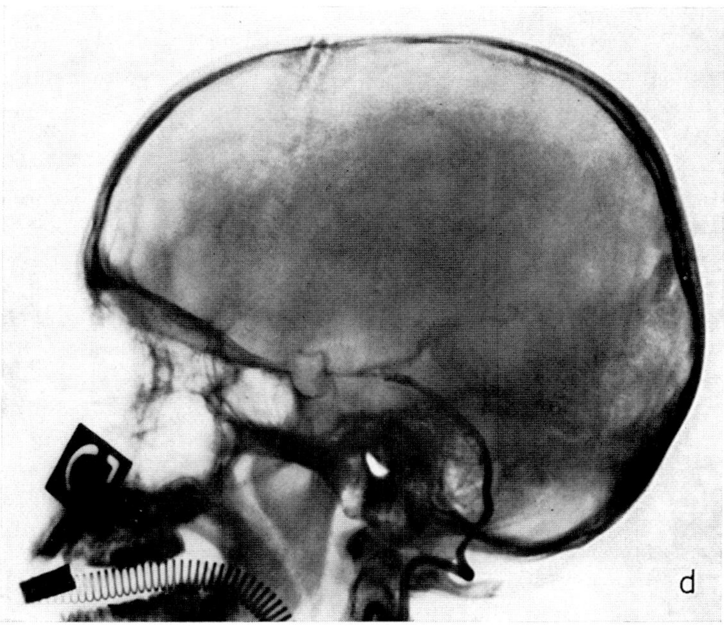

Fig. 25d

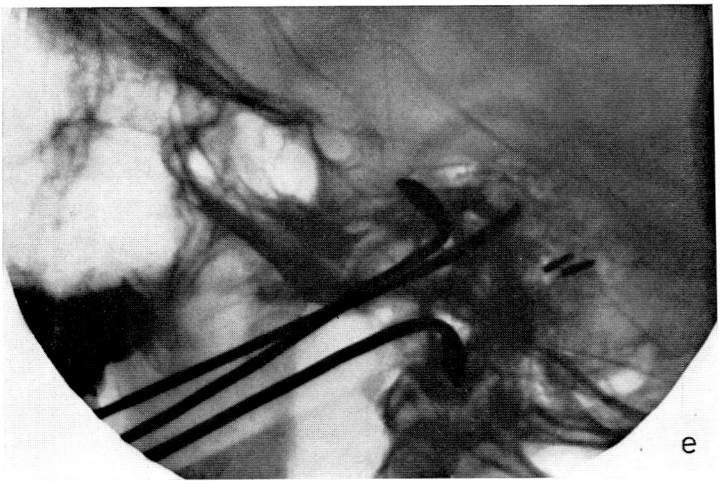

Fig. 25e

Fig. 25. Association of transoral and intradural approaches in two stages. a) and b) Chordoma partially calcified in a 10 years old boy, with a dorso clival destruction (the tumor does not overlap the spheno-occipital synchondrosis). c) and d) Deformation of vertebral and basilar arteries. e) Intra-operative radiography during the transoral approach showing the limits of removal. Clips are on the dura. One month after the intra-dural remnants of the tumor were removed through a subtemporal and sub-occipital route

lateral extension of the tumor towards the pterygoids, or the lesser or greater sphenoid wings, and middle fossa, or when the tumor invades most of the clival area from the sphenoid body to the foramen magnum or upper cervical spine (Fig. 24).

c) Combined Approaches in One Stage

The case described in Figs. 22 a, b, c, d, e, and f is a good example of a combined procedure. The patient had had a previous incomplete removal of a chordoma via a transphenoidal route. Three years later it was necessary to reoperate. At this time, the patient presented with drop attacks, and on X-rays, the tumor was found to be partially calcified. A combined, single stage transphenoidal-transbasal procedure was used. Gross total removal of the tumor was accomplished, The patient is doing well 7 years later. Two others have benefited from this same procedure. In another case (Fig. 23), a transbasal approach was combined with a "pseudo" transoral route. The softness of the posterior pharyngeal wall permitted in this case the manual milking of the tumor, backwards, into the operative field afforded by a transbasal procedure, without opening the pharyngeal mucosa.

d) Combined Approaches in Multiple Stages

Some cases of very large chordomas extending both intra and extra cranially are not amenable to complete resection by one single approach.

The intradural exposures do not permit the resection of the invaded bone, and it may be anticipated that extradural approaches could result in dural tears and cerebrospinal leaks. In such cases, in the absence of raised intracranial pressure, extradural attack on the tumor may be performed 2 or 3 months before the remainder of the lesion is approached intradurally. This is illustrated in Figs. 24 a, b, c, d, and e. Subtemporal removal of the interpeduncular remnant of a large tumor resected 2 months previously by an extradural approach was carried out. The large bony defect left by the initial resection had been previously repaired by bone grafts. In the case demonstrated in Figs. 25 a, b, c, d, and e, gross complete tumor removal was accomplished via a subtemporal and subtentorial resection, preceded 1 month earlier by a transoral procedure. Unfortunately, the patient developed a pharyngeal cerebrospinal fluid leak, meningitis and died, as a consequence of a wound of the pharyngeal mucosa by introducing a nasogastric tube. Such an event should always be kept in mind. It stresses the fragility of the pharyngeal scar.

IV. Conclusion

Other surgical procedures may eventually be designed to cope with tumors of the base of the skull. The recently developed transbasal approach permits a more radical and complete ablation of neoplasms in the sphenoidal and clival areas. Other approaches may be used depending on the topography and the type of the tumor, as specified in this paper. Several routes may be combined in one or multiple stages. The neurosurgeon must be aware of these procedures, and must be ready to apply them when the need arises.

References

1. Derome, P. J., Trigo, J. C., 1966: Mucocèles et empyèmes du sinus sphénoïdal. (Rev. Neurol. *115*, 980—983.)
2. Derome, P. J., *et al.*, 1972: Les tumeurs sphéno-ethmoïdales ; Possibilités d'exérèse et de réparation chirurgicales. Rapport de la Société de Neuro-Chirurgie de Langue Française. Neuro-chirurgie *15*, Suppl. 1, 1—164.
3. Derome, P. J., 1977: The transbasal approach to tumors invading the base of the skull. In: Currents Techniques in Operative Neurosurgery, pp. 223—245, edited by H. H. Schmidek and W. H. Sweet. New York: Grune and Stratton.
4. Falconer, M. A., Bailey, I. C., Duchen, L. N., 1968: Surgical treatment of chordoma and chondroma of the skull base. J. Neurosurg. *29*, 261—275.
5. Geissenger, J. D., Siqueira, E. B., Ross, E. R., 1970: Giant cell tumors of the sphenoid bone. J. Neurosurg. *32*, 665—670.
6. Guiot, G., Derome, P. J., 1966: A propos des méningiomes en plaque du ptérion. Le traitement chirurgical des méningiomes osseux hyperostosants. Ann. Chir. *20*, 19—20: C 1109—C 1127.
7. Krayenbühl, H., Yaşargil, M. G., 1975: Chondromas. Progr. neurol. Surg. *6*, 435—463 (Basel: Karger).
8. Krayenbühl, H., Yaşargil, M. G., 1975: Cranial chordomas. Progr. neurol. Surg. *6*, 380—434 (Basel: Karger).
9. Laine, E., Delandsheer, J. M., Jomin, M., *et al.*, 1977: Indications et possibilités de la voie transbuccopharyngée. Neuro-chirurgie *23*, 249—314.
10. Pertuiset, B., Beciric, T., 1958: La voie intracranienne dans l'exérèse du prolongement nasal des méningiomes olfactifs. Press. Med. *63*, 1863—1865.

11. Rougerie, J., Guiot, G., Bouche, J., Trigo, J. C., 1967: Les voies d'abord du chordome du clivus. Neuro-chirurgie *13*, 559—570.
12. Saunders, W. H., Miglets, A., 1967: Surgical techniques for eradicating far advanced carcinoma of the orbital ethmoid and maxillary areas. Trans. Am. Acad. Ophthalmol. Otolaryngol. *7*, 426—431.
13. Stevenson, G. C., Stoney, R. J., Perkins, R. K., Adams, J. R., 1966: A transcervical, transclival approach to the ventral surface of the brainstem for removal of a clivus chordoma. J. Neurosurg. *24*, 544—551.
14. Tessier, P., Guiot, G., Derome, P. J., 1973: Orbital hypertelorism. II: Definite treatment of orbital hypertelorism by craniofacial or by extracranial osteotomies. Scand. Plast. Reconstr. Surg. *7*, 39—58.
15. Van Buren, J. M., Ommaya, A. K., Ketcham, A. S., 1968: Ten year's experience with radical combined cranio-facial resection of malignant tumors of the paranasal sinuses. J. Neurosurg. *28*, 341—350.

Cervical Spondylotic Myelopathy

R. Braakman

Neurosurgical Department, Academic Hospital Dijkzigt, Erasmus University, Rotterdam (The Netherlands)

With 17 Figures

Contents

Cervical spondylotic myelopathy is the most common disease of the spinal cord after the age of 40. There have been many publications advocating various types of surgical treatment, and their results, on the basis of relatively small and selected series of patients with spondylotic myelopathy. Opinions about the preferable approach vary. There is not as yet full knowledge regarding the pathomechanism of the disease and the factors governing its natural course. However, it is clear that mechanical factors play an important role. This means that most surgical therapies have a mechanical basis. These surgical approaches are on the whole not difficult technically; the main problem is the best choice for each individual patient.

This paper does not provide an answer to this problem; it summarizes current views and is intended as a guideline for a more rational choice and a flexible surgical strategy.

Spondylotic Myelopathy

Spondylotic Myelopathy (SM) has some characteristic clinical features. These features commonly include: gait disturbance, weakness and stiffness of the legs, spastic weakness of the upper extremities, impaired postural sensibility of the legs and various sensory disturbances of the arms. These features, however, are not pathognomic for SM and may occur in various other diseases. The diagnosis SM is made largely by exclusion of other neurological disorders with related signs such as motor neurone disease, syringomyelia, spinal tumors, subacute combined degeneration of the cord and multiple sclerosis. Multiple sclerosis and spondylotic myelopathy may coexist (Brain and Wilkinson 1957).

It is wise to remember that Hughes (1966) established that at post mortem of 20 patients whose diagnosis was SM, only eight had the disease, 6 others had multiple sclerosis and/or arteriosclerotic cord disease, one a meningioma and 5 spondylosis with a trauma.

A detailed description of the various syndromes which may occur in SM and the considerations to differentiate the clinical features from those of the other diseases are beyond the scope of this chapter. The reader is referred to *e.g.:* Brain *et al.* 1952, Clarke and Robinson 1956, Brain and Wilkinson 1967, Adams 1977, Robinson *et al.* 1977.

Definition

Not every cord disease due to an affection of the spine is properly called spondylotic myelopathy. The designation SM is commonly not used in cord involvement due to diseases of the spine like rheumatoid arthritis, congenital anomalies, injuries, recent disc protrusions and tumours. However, the recently reported ossification of posterior longitudinal ligaments—particularly occurring in the Japanese (Ono *et al.* 1977) is commonly included as a separate cause of SM.

Spondylosis

The term cervical spondylosis comprises all degenerative changes of the cervical spine. Spondylosis occurs particularly between C_3 and C_7, either at a single site, *e.g.* as a late reaction to a disc protrusion or—more commonly—as a diffuse disorder. Early spondylosis is characterized by lateral bending and elongation of the uncinate processes and by gradual narrowing of the intervertebral space. With advancing age and degeneration the intervertebral discs lose their ability to retain water under high pressure. Subsequently tears in the anulus develop, the fibres of the anulus hyalinize and the height of the disc diminishes. The endplates of the vertebral bodies lose there concavity and their bony structure condenses. Osteophytes are formed at the end of the vertebral bodies. They may occur in the midline or only in the uncovertebral region and may also involve the whole posterior aspect of the vertebral body (Fig. 1). Elongation of the uncinate processes and lipping impinge on the anterior wall of the intervertebral canal. Usually the C_5–C_6 and C_6–C_7 discs are involved first and spurs occur particularly

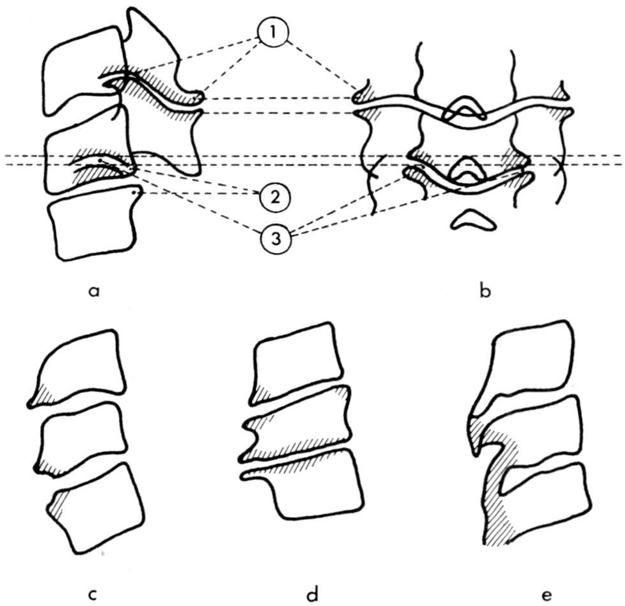

Fig. 1. Schematic representations of the most significant spondylotic changes of the lower cervical spine. a) and b) show intervertebral arthrosis deformans (*1*) and uncovertebral osteochondrosis (*2*) in lateral and AP projection. The uncovertebral fissures ("joint" spaces, *3*) are visible on the lateral projection because of the eversion of the uncinate processes. The osteophytes seen at the posterior margins of the vertebral end-plates (*2*) as a rule are medially localized uncovertebral osteophytes. c) Schmorl's spondylosis deformans. d) Flattening of a vertebral body with spondylosis deformans. e) Ankylosing vertebral hyperostosis

on both sides of these discs. As a reaction to disc degeneration the adjoining vertebral bodies may decrease in height and elongate in sagittal direction.

Retrolisthesis, dorsal displacement of a vertebral body in relation with its caudal neighbour, is particularly seen in deflexion at the C_3–C_4 and C_4–C_5 level. It may be due to a large range of movement in the corresponding motor-segment, but may also be the result of disc degeneration.

As a result of these various phenomena, the sagittal diameter of the spinal canal diminishes.

Spondylosis may also lead to a change of the spinal curvature, often resulting in a low cervical kyphosis.

Arthrosis of the intervertebral (zygapophysial) joint narrows the joint space and leads to eburnation of the articular surfaces. Here too, additional bone is formed. These spurs usually narrow the intervertebral canal on the posterior aspect, whereas narrowing on the anterior wall is the result of uncovertebral spurs (Fig. 1). Spondylotic and arthrotic changes usually start to become visible radiologically after the age of 40 and can be detected in over 50% of radiographs in people of 50 years of age and more (Brooker and Barter 1965, Friedenberg and Miller 1963, Pallis *et al.* 1954, Penning 1968).

Pathological Mechanism

The presence of cervical spondylosis in a patient with the clinical features of SM is insufficient to establish the spondylosis as the cause of the clinical features, despite the fact that no one without spondylosis develops SM (Robinson *et al.* 1977). There is poor correlation between the amount of spondylotic change on the radiographs and the degree of neurological deficit. There is also no correlation between the rate of growth of the osteophytes and the rate of clinical deterioration. These facts mark the main problems of SM: the diagnosis and the pathogenesis of the disease.

If there is little relation between SM and the degree of spondylosis, what then is the cause of cord involvement in cervical spondylosis? The pathogenesis seems to be by no means stereotyped for all cases (Crandall and Gregorius 1977).

Arnold (1955) and Mayfield (1955) established that in cases with SM the average width of the lower cervical canal is about 3 mm less than in cases of spondylosis without myelopathy. This was confirmed by others (Adams and Logue 1971, Burrows 1963, Nurick 1972, Wilkinson *et al.* 1969).

These findings support the proponents of a mechanical cause who ascribe the cord involvement to recurrent minor traumata.

In this mechanical concept the myelopathy is the result of either:

a. Compression of the cord in sagittal direction, particularly through a "pincers grip" mechanism, that is compression of the cord from both sides (Penning and van der Zwaag 1964, Adams 1976).

b. Pathologically increased tension and overstretching of the cord in anteflexion over the spondylotic ridges, resulting in pressure from one side: "contactpressure" (Breig 1960, Breig and El-Nadi 1966).

ad a. The sagittal diameter of the spinal canal shows large variations between individuals. The upper limit may have a value up to 70% more than the lower one (Boysen 1954, Burrows 1963, Penning 1968, Wolf *et al.* 1956). This diameter is in mobile spines usually significantly less in extension[1] than in flexion due to the sliding movements of the vertebra on its caudal partner (Fig. 2). In extension the cord shortens and thickens,

[1] Some authors prefer to use the terms flexion and extension for forward and backward bending of head and neck, others prefer anteflexion and deflexion or retroflexion. In this chapter the first of the two alternatives is used.

but the sagittal diameter does not vary so much between individuals (Burrows 1963, Nugent 1959). This means that the space around the cord—the "play" of the cord—(Penning 1968) within the bony spinal canal shows important individual variations, particularly in the lower cervical part of the canal. In subjects with a naturally large diameter of the canal and consequently of the subarachnoid space, the spinal cord has more free play than in individuals with a natural small diameter in which the cord may be caught in a "tight fit". This is particularly the case in extension. Whether or not cord compression occurs depends on the degree of movement of the spine and the amount of space available in the spinal canal for the spinal cord and on how much is left for innocuous encroachment (Hinck and

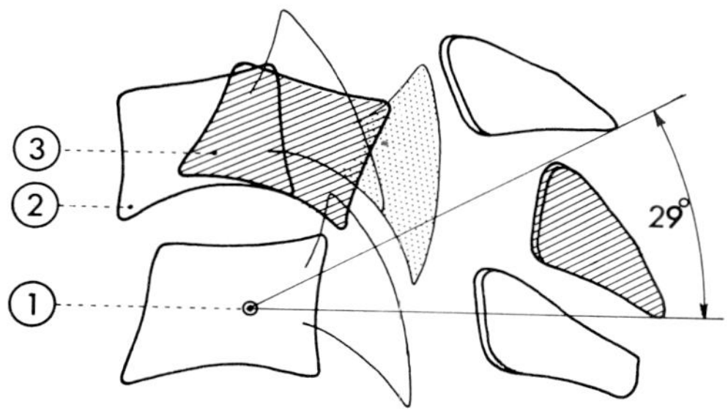

Fig. 2. Diagrams of flexion-extension movement in the lower cervical motor segments. Two types of movement diagrams indicating the relative movement in the sagittal plane between two lower cervical vertebrae. Total range of movement: 29°. *1* Motor axis. *2* Flexed position of the mobile vertebra. *3* Extended position of the mobile vertebra. Note that the sagittal diameter of the spinal canal—between postero-inferior part of the upper vertebral body and arch of the lower vertebra—is less in extension than it is in flexion

Sachdev 1966). Any degree of intervertebral disc protrusion, adjacent osteophytic overgrowth or—perhaps—swelling of the non-bony soft tissues like buckled hypertrophic ligamenta flava (Nurick 1972, Taylor 1953) will diminish the functional sagittal diameter of the canal.

If the spinal canal is small by nature, relatively little encroachment by osteophytes, vertebral retrolisthesis or ligamenta flava can be tolerated without causing spinal cord compression. This means that compression of the cord occurs sooner in a shallow canal with a small protrusion or local retrolisthesis.

However, in a wide canal compression may also occur when there are extremely large protrusions. The level of the pinching in sagittal direction is sometimes the level of maximum growths of osteophytes (usually C_5–C_6, C_6–C_7) but in many cases it is the level where in extension the retrolisthesis occurs, which is usually C_3–C_4 or C_4–C_5. The cord is then compressed between the body of the retrolisthetic vertebra and the arch of the underlying neighbour (Fig. 3, 4, 5).

ad b. In flexion the cord is stretched and is situated against the anterior border of the canal. This may be uneven, particularly in elderly persons

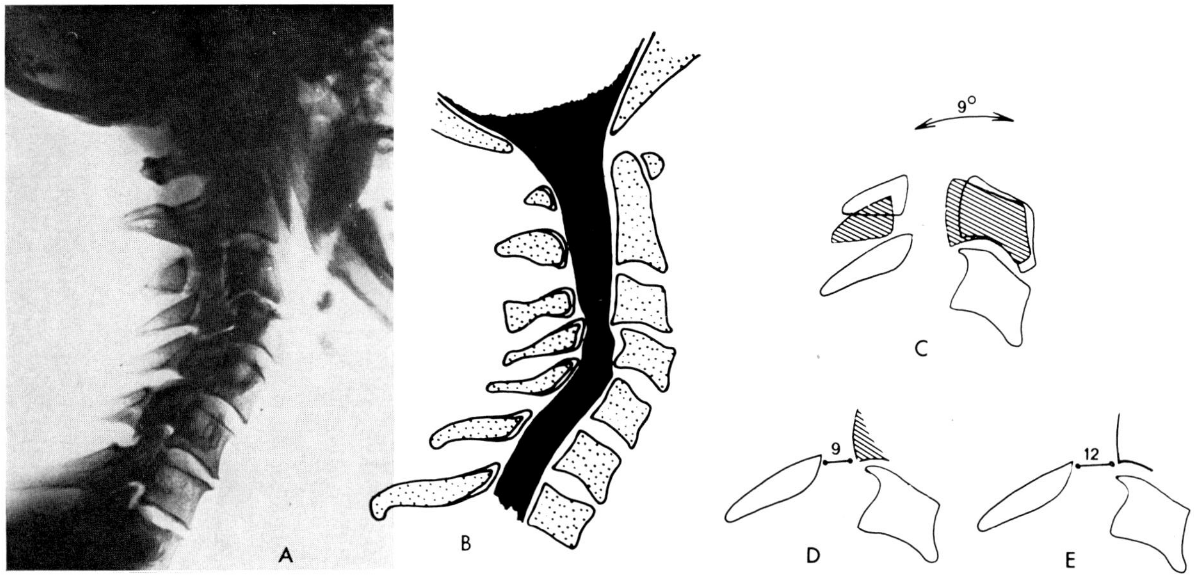

Fig. 3. The effect of pincers mechanism, responsible for compression of the spinal cord in extension of the neck. Forty-six-year old male with spastic tetraparesis. A) Lateral radiograph of the cervical spine showing C_3–C_4 retrolisthesis. Naturally narrow spinal canal. B) Drawing of the radiograph. C) Movement diagram of C_3–C_4 made on the basis of D) and E). Sagittal diameter of the bony canal: in extension 9 mm and in flexion 12 m m

due to bulging of discs and spondylotic ridges. In flexion the length of the anterior border of the bony canal increases up to 13 per cent and the posterior border up to 70 per cent. The cord adapts itself to this varying length of the canal. It follows the shortest route through the canal, apparently as a result of its elastic tension (Fig. 6 a–e). This may result in pathologically increased tension and overstretching of the cord in flexion

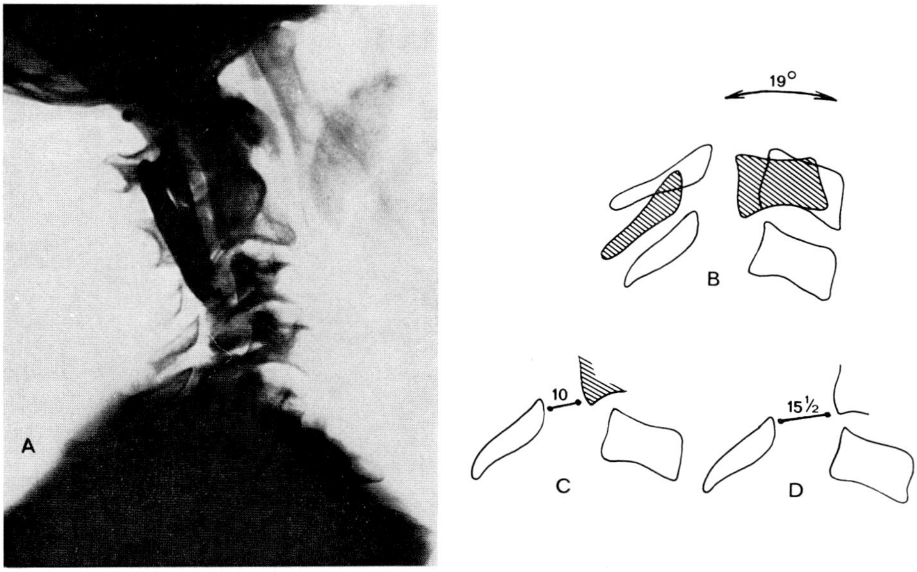

Fig. 4. 55-year-old male with myelopathy of three years' duration. A) Ethiodan myelogram. The suboccipitally injected contrast medium is arrested at C_3–C_4. B) Motor diagram of C_3–C_4. Range of movement 19°. Considerable narrowing of the spinal canal in extension. C) and D) Separate views of the jaw of the bony pincers in extension and flexion with a diameter of 10 and 15,5 mm respectively

over the spondylotic ridges, particularly in those spines which—in mid-position—show already low cervical kyphosis as a result of disc degeneration.

The controversial issue whether the cord moves up and down during movement (Breig 1960, Reid 1960) seems to be decisively solved by the experiments of Adams and Logue (1971). They showed that cord and dura move up and down particularly when there are descending extrathecal roots. This means that during motion there may be not only pressure on the cord but also friction.

In each individual case the most appropriate operation is the one which abolishes the most important of each of these pathological factors.

However, even in cases of SM in which pinching of the cord can be demonstrated symptoms often do not disappear after adequate laminectomy. This means that other causes may also play a role.

Kahn (1947) *e.g.* stated that the dentate ligaments held the cord against the spondylotic ridges. For decades these ligaments were cut during operations. Reid (1960), Aboulker *et al.* (1965) and Stoltman and Blackwood (1964) showed that dividing the dentate ligaments did not influence the degree of contact between cord and protrusions, even in flexion. Aboulker *et al.* (1965) showed by postoperative myelography in patients after laminectomy in whom the dentate ligaments were not cut, that decompression

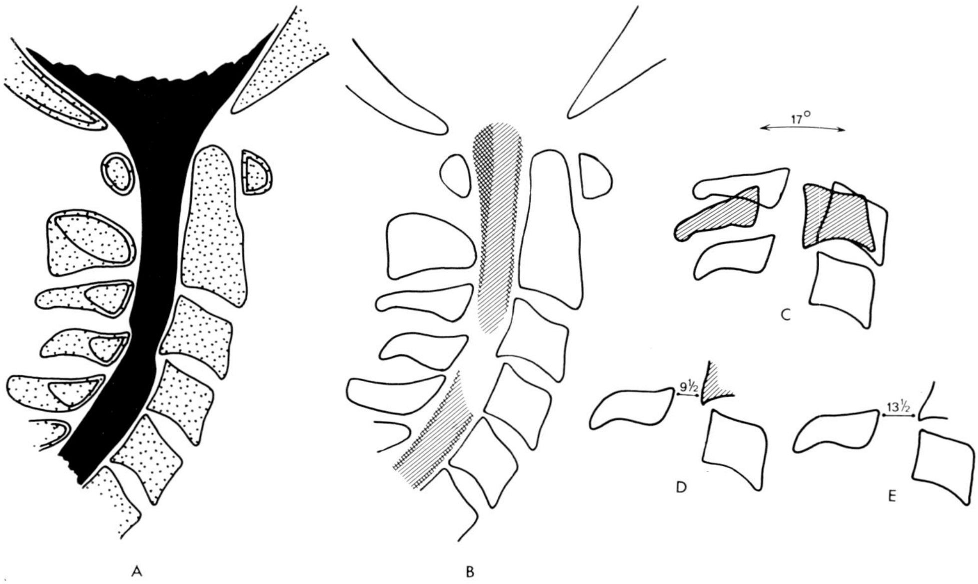

Fig. 5. 53-year-old female with a retrolisthesis C_3–C_4 and only minimal osteophytes. A) Drawing of the lateral radiograph with supposed configuration of the dural sac. B) Drawing of the myelogram with the complete block in extension at the C_3–C_4 level. C) Movement diagram. Range of movement: 17°. D) Diameter in extension 9,5 mm. E) Diameter in flexion 13,5 mm

was obtained in all cases with posterior transposition of the cord and with the appearance of a perimedullary space anteriorly and posteriorly.

Adams and Logue (1971) established that more severe symptoms were found in those patients who had more than average extension movement and fewer in those with more flexion movement, even although the total amount of neck motion was about equal in both groups. According to Gonzalez-Feria (1975) and Aboulker (1965) laminectomy itself may induce a new pathogenetic factor: the post-operative connective tissue scar. They showed that in flexion sometimes the sagittal diameter between the vertebral body and the scar is 6 mm or less, suggesting recurrent cord compression by the scar, particularly in flexion. Various authors (Clarke and Robinson 1956, Nurick 1972) attributed significance to arachnoidal adhesions. These adhesions no doubt exist in many cases of SM, but we believe that these are secondary reactions to the above mentioned factors.

Taylor (1964) thought that the variability and diffuseness of the symptoms in SM was most reasonably explained by intermittent vascular interruption. Many authors agreed but held different views regarding the site of this interruption. The interference was by many supposed to be localized in the intervertebral canals through tethering of the nerve root sleeves (Adams and Logue 1971) with consequent interference in the blood flow during neck motion or through pressure by large osteophytes. Palleske (1970) and Gooding and Wilson (1978) believe that this results in arterial spasm and in episodic loss of autoregulation.

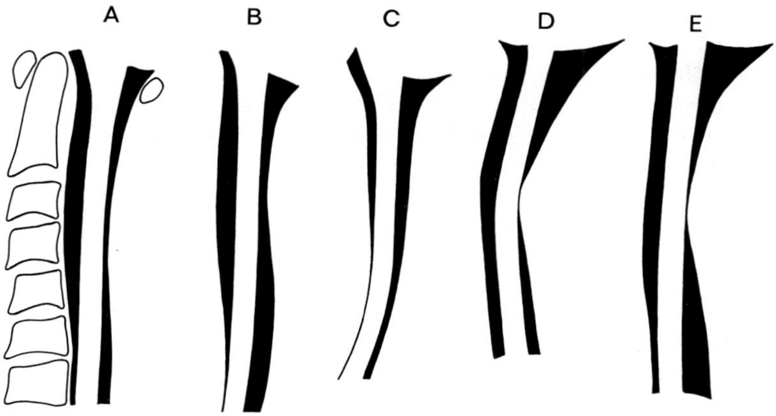

Fig. 6. Position of the spinal cord in several cervical spines, as recorded from myelograms in cadavers. Note that the cord always follows the shortest route through the spinal canal. The regions of contact between the cord and the anterior or posterior border of the spinal canal depend on the particular configuration of the canal

Others localize the cause in the anterior spinal artery (Mair and Druckmann 1953), the border line area between anterior spinal artery and posterior spinal artery (Tönnis 1961, Zülch 1954) the perimedullary arteries (Shimomura and Hukuda 1968), the intrinsic vascular supply in the cord itself through pressure of the cord against osteophytes and associated distortion (Breig *et al.* 1966) or in the veins leading to congestion and later embarrassment of the arterial supply (Brain and Wilkinson 1967, Gillilan 1970).

With the present state of knowledge such supposed vascular factors can hardly be influenced even by foraminotomy. Adhesions, if cut, usually recur. This means that the emphasis of therapy should be on the abolition of mechanical factors.

Additional Investigations

The aim of all additional investigation in any case of suspected SM is to exclude other diseases with related symptoms and to define a plausible cause for the cord involvement. This may then result in a rational basis for therapy.

Radiology

The aim of radiological procedures is to demonstrate compression, particularly pinching of the cord in sagittal direction at one or more levels or to provide support for the assumption that pathologically increased axial tension may be present. Attention should not be focused on the radiological "severity" of spondylosis, but on the reduction of the available room for the spinal cord to move, and in its freedom of movement, together with any possible contact pressure on the cord. In any patient with suspected SM radiographs should include lateral, anteroposterior and oblique views; plain films will reveal possible bony impingements on the spinal cord, but only myelography will reveal whether or not this is present.

On the lateral radiographs the presence or absence of spondylotic changes and their influence on the spinal canal should be noted. Medial and lateral —*i.e.* unconvertebral—spurs may overlap. Midline or paramedian spurs may be the cause of myelopathy, lateral spurs may be an indication of root involvement. To distinguish the two types of spurs AP, right and left oblique views may be helpful, but perfect lateral tomograms are indispensable and these tomograms should preferably be taken with the neck in extension. On these lateral radiographs the *natural* and *functional* sagittal diameter should be measured. A marker of *e.g.* 5 cm length should be temporarily fixed to the skin of the neck in the midline as reference for measurements.

The *natural* diameter is measured between the midpart of the posterior aspect of the vertebral body and the nearest point of the arch, *i.e.* the junction of the arch of that vertebra with the spinous process (Burrows 1963). The mean natural diameter at the C_3–C_7 level is 17 mm $\pm$ 5 (Boysen 1954, Burrows 1963, Nurick 1972, Penning 1962) and 2,25 mm less in the Japanese (Murone 1974). There is thus a wide variation between individuals.

The minimal *functional* sagittal diameter—from a ridge or a retrolisthetic body to the closest posterior bony landmark—usually occurs in extension. It is often at the level of a retrolisthesis, but may also be at the level of the most marked spondylotic ridges or adjacent to block-vertebrae. Bony pinching of the cord is almost certain when the sagittal diameter of the bony canal is 10 mm or less (real value) at one or more sites. Pinching is possible when the diameter is 10 to 12 mm and highly improbable with a diameter of 13 mm or more (Symon and Lavender 1967).

The fact that the cord follows the shortest route through the spinal canal means that even with the lower part of the spine in flexion, the cord may in certain cases be in contact with the posterior border of the canal at a higher level depending on the peculiar form of the individual spine (Fig. 6 e). Therefore, before any surgical procedure is started, a drawing should be made of the supposed position of the cord in the canal on plain films in flexion and in extension, to reveal the sites of contact with the anterior and posterior border.

Oblique views—taken to display foramina—should be interpreted with caution. Often foramina are not exactly parallel to each other. In our experience it is not uncommon that the diagnosis narrowing of a foramen is made, when the foramina are not well displayed, due to slight rotation in one motor segment or an imprecise radiographic projection. This may give rise to error. The diagnosis of narrowing of a foramen is permissible only if noticeable uncovertebral or arthrotic spurs can be demonstrated beyond any doubt.

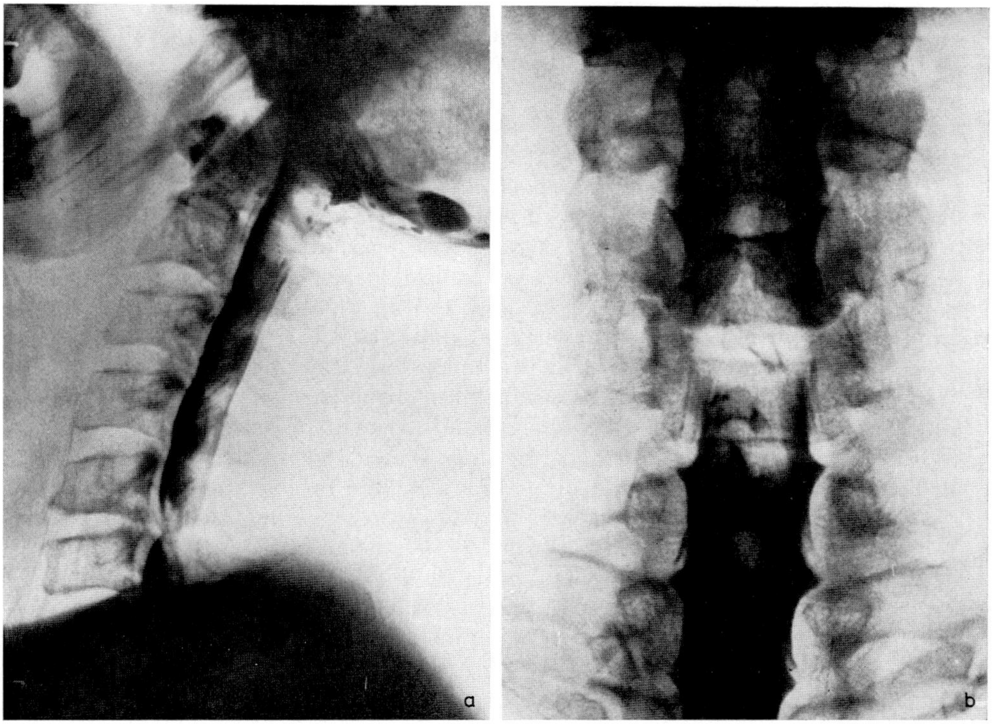

Fig. 7. Slowly progressive mild cord signs in a 43 year old patient. Plain radiography reveals small posterior osteophytes at the C_5–C_6 level. The spinal canal is of normal size. Lumbar puncture: normal CSF; normal manometry. Tomographic metrizamide myelography (a, b) displays a more than expected anterior compression of the cord at the C_5–C_6 level (C_6–C_7 not well visible; but was normal). This is a case for an anterior approach and *e.g.* either a Robinson and Smith fusion, or a Cloward approach with removal of osteophytes and disc extrusion and subsequent dowel fusion

Contrastprocedures

Myelopathy is often the result of bony impingement but may also be due to soft tissue changes. On plain radiographs osteophytes may show up very little and appear to be much smaller than in fact they are. These additional changes in the spinal canal may be visualized through radiographic contrastprocedures (Fig. 7). In cases with obvious bony pinching of the cord myelography provides only occasionally additional diagnostic important information. Myelography is, however, mandatory if there is any doubt about the diagnosis. It can then exclude other causes, such as an unexpected extramedullary tumor.

Until a few years ago the choice between oily contrast and air was an important issue. The advantage of oil is that the presence of pulsatile movements and the passage of the contrast medium can be examined fluoroscopically and checked in various positions of the spine. Oily contrast allows a functional investigation. In case of multiple narrowings, however, the contrast column is commonly broken into parts and the information obtained is usually already available on the plain functional radiographs. With oil the diameter of the cord in the sagittal plane and its situation in the spinal canal cannot be sufficiently appreciated. Midline invaginations are easily missed, because the contrast pools in the lateral gutters (Crandall and Gregorius 1977, Heinz and Goldman 1972).

With gas and tomograms the position of the cord and its diameter can be well visualized. It is, however, a lengthy, rather invasive and unpleasant procedure with the possibility of faulty interpretation. Much technical expertise is required to align the longitudinal axis of the canal with the tomographic cut (Crandall and Hanafee 1964). Functional myelography is impossible and the demonstration of a diminution of pulsatile movements in certain positions *e.g.* extension is impossible. The introduction of amipaque (metrizamide) means an important improvement, it produces an image of the cord and fills the entire canal. It is at present the best choice available. This kind of myelography may reveal protrusions obviously not of bony nature, which are not detectable on plain radiographs.

The findings during vertebral angiography in spondylosis have been reported by Penning 1968 and Verbiest 1972. The examination does not provide additional information in patients with myelopathy, but may be indicated if surgical treatment of spondylotic radiculopathy is considered.

We have no experience with spinal phlebography; this procedure may not be as easy to perform as in the lumbar area and its usefulness is not established in the cervical region.

Discograms are of extremely doubtful diagnostic and localizing value in patients with myelopathy (Holt 1964).

Lumbar Puncture

Support for the presence of compression of the cord can be obtained through lumbar puncture with manometric studies in various positions of the neck (Kaplan and Kennedy 1950). A block during postural manometry reveals obstruction to the CSF pathways, but does not necessarily imply compression of the cord. The same holds true for a myelographic block. Both blocks prove that the cord is clasped between the walls of the spinal canal, but the degree of compression can not be predicted. Radiological diagnosis of cord compression becomes highly probable, however, in case of narrowing of the canal to 10 mm or less, combined with a complete obstruction of the CSF pathways as judged by manometry or myelography. This combination is strongly suggestive of spondylotic cord compression being the cause of the myelopathy (Adams 1976, Clarke and Robinson 1956, Lakke 1969).

Normal manometry in various positions of the neck is rare in SM, but does occur, particularly in patients with a change in the spinal curvature. In most cases of SM the protein content of the CSF is normal or mildly elevated (Clarke and Robinson 1956) usually not more than 100 mg% (Adams 1976). Elevated gammaglobulin levels on the contrary, suggest multiple sclerosis and a high protein content is an indication of a tumor.

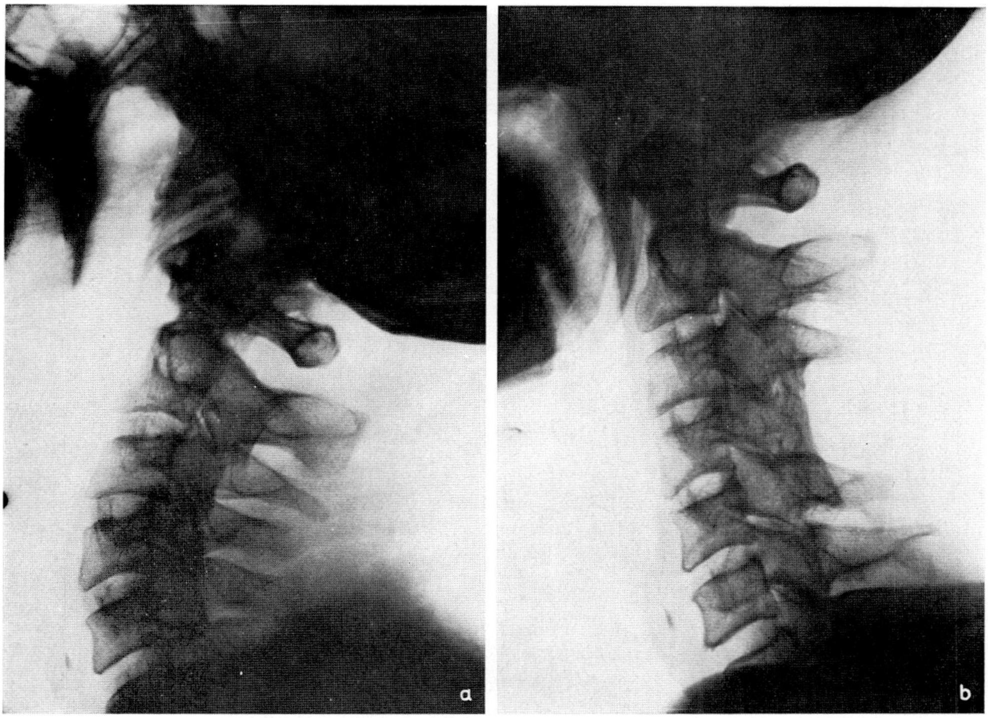

Fig. 8. This 46 year old man with a retrolisthesis C_3–C_4 (a) got a central cord lesion after an extension injury. The neurosurgeon in charge performed laminectomy C_4 and a postlateral fusion, which was meant as a preventive measure against recurrence (b). Complete neurologic recovery. Optimal fusion. The present author prefers to treat these patients conservatively and would in this patient not have performed a preventive laminectomy and fusion as such a procedure carries the risk of an increase in cord signs. He considers the operation indicated only in those rare cases in which the expected rate of recovery with conservative treatment (depending upon the type of cord syndrome) does not occur or in the very rare case of late progressive cord lesion

Neither laminectomy nor fusion procedures should be undertaken without lumbar puncture for manometric studies and c.s.f. examination. If manometry is normal, the value of laminectomy in particular may be questioned as patients with a block seem to react better to laminectomy than those without (Gonzalez-Feria and Peraita-Peraita 1975, Lakke 1969).

Trauma

Repeated minor traumata are generally considered to be one of the main causes of SM. However, one major injury, particularly those resulting in extension of the neck, may give the same pincers grip of the cord, often with more disastrous effect as in many cases a total or severe incomplete tetraplegia may ensue. In incomplete cord lesions the clinical syndrome is usually a central cord lesion.

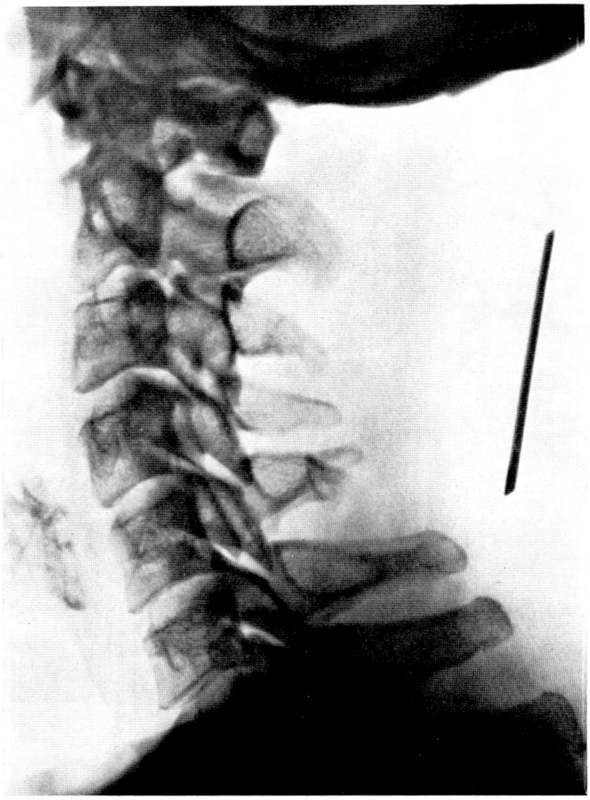

Fig. 9. Girl 18 years, fell from her bicycle. Complete tetraplegia! Note the natural shallowness of the canal, predisposing to a severe cord lesion after a relatively minor injury. The sagittal diameter of the canal at C_5 is 9 mm in the midline. The marker in the nape of the neck has a length of 5 cm

In most cases there is no permanent misalignment of the cervical spine and radiographs do not display signs of traumatic damage to the spine. In many textbooks of neurology these cases—usually involving patients over 40 years of age—are described under the heading: haematomyelia. These radiographs commonly show, however, marked spondylosis and/or a narrow sagittal diameter of the spinal canal (Alexander *et al.* 1958, Braakman and Penning 1971, Schneider 1969) (Fig. 8, 9). In our opinion, the relative weakness of the intervertebral disc is an important contributary

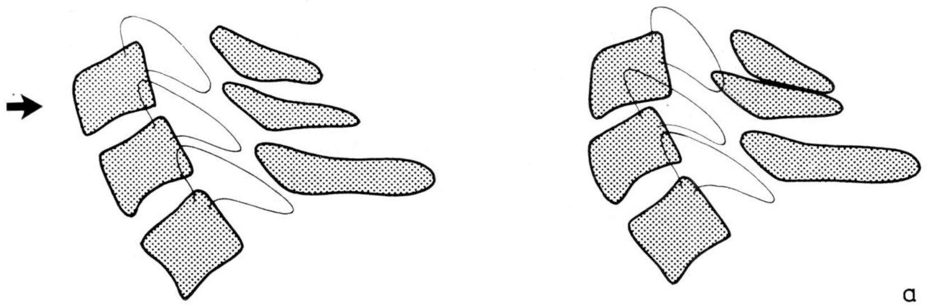

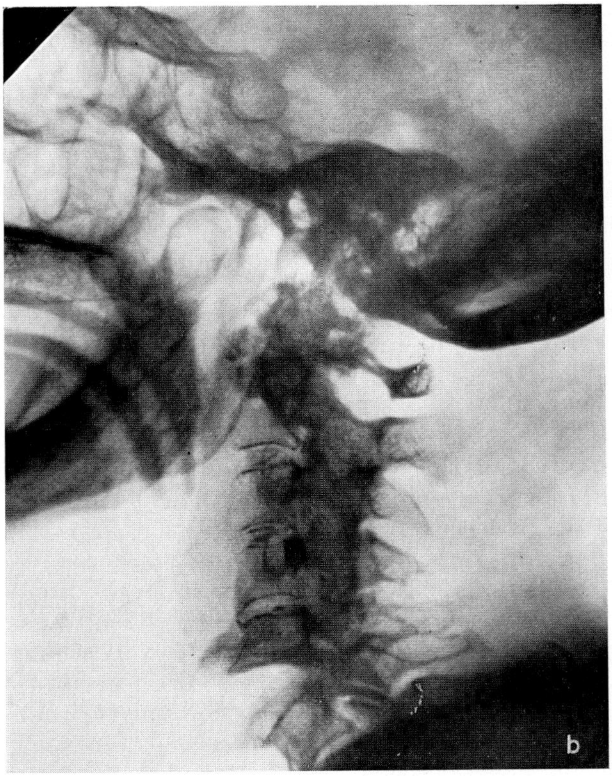

Fig. 10. Mechanism in case of traumatic cord lesion without radiological signs of traumatic involvement of the spine. Due to disc degeneration with a bisected disc the anterior longitudinal ligament ruptures easily and the cranial vertebra can move backwards in relation to its caudal neighbour even after relatively mild injuries (a). This causes a pincers grip of the cord particularly when the natural sagittal diameter of the spinal canal is small or when there are marked osteophytes on the postero-inferior side of the vertebral body. After the injury the alignment is commonly restored. Occasionally however, the lateral radiograph on admission of the patient displays the damage to anterior longitudinal ligament and disc (b)

factor in the genesis of these hyperextension injuries of the spinal cord, especially in cases in which it has been completely bisected by the spondylotic process. Since the anterior longitudinal ligament is not supported by the cohesive strength of the disc, it ruptures easily. This will result in significant displacement of the vertebral bodies and consequent pinching of the spinal cord between the temporarily posteriorly displaced vertebral body and the arch of its caudal neighbour. Braakman and Penning (1971) designate these traumatic cases as "hyperextension sprains" (Fig. 10). The diagnosis is mostly based on the severity of the neurological picture in the absence of radiological signs, supported incidentally by clinical evidence such as the history of the accident and the presence of wounds of the jaws, face, forehead, throat etc. Hyperextension of the neck to display the tearing of the anterior longitudinal ligament and disc should not be performed "in vivo" because of the danger of pinching the cord again. In doubtful cases calcification of the anterior side of the disc, a few years after the accident, may provide a vital clue to the diagnosis (Braakman and Penning 1971).

In elderly patients with spondylosis or in younger patients with a natural small diameter of the cervical canal manipulative hyperextension of the neck during intubation, tonsillectomy and tooth-extraction may also result in spinal cord lesions (Symonds 1953).

Therapy

In most pathogenetic concepts, movements of the spine, particularly flexion or extension play an important role, either by induction of pinching or pathological axial tension of the cord, or through intermittent compression of radicular vessels.

The call for surgical intervention is the more urgent when the natural course, with or without conservative therapeutic measures, leads to progressive decline. There is unfortunately insufficient information about the natural course of SM without surgical intervention as patients with more severe or progressive involvement of the cord are commonly operated upon. Clarke and Robinson (1956) state that in most patients progression is in episodes and in the minority steady and slow. Some cases are according to them definitely progressive after an injury and it is unusual for spontaneous regression to occur. Robinson *et al.* (1977) confirms that 20% of their cases showed steady slow progression and only 5% a rapid onset of symptoms after which no new features appeared. In their series too a complete remission never occurred.

There is no doubt that immobilization of the neck with a brace or bedrest may result in temporary improvement of the complaints in legs and arms, particularly in those cases with a high range of movement of the neck in the sagittal plane (Bradshaw 1957, Clarke and Robinson 1956, Lees and Turner 1963, Robinson *et al.* 1977, Teng 1960).

After removal of the brace signs usually, but not always, recur. Longlasting external immobilization of the neck is hardly ever tolerated by nonneurotic individuals.

Surgical Therapy

There are many surgical approaches, all meant to abolish the supposed causative factor of SM. This may be either through laminectomy or by anterior transdiscal or lateral removal of the spurs on the anterior side of the cord. Both approaches may be combined with anterior or posterior fusion procedures. Neither the anterior approach nor laminectomy elimi-

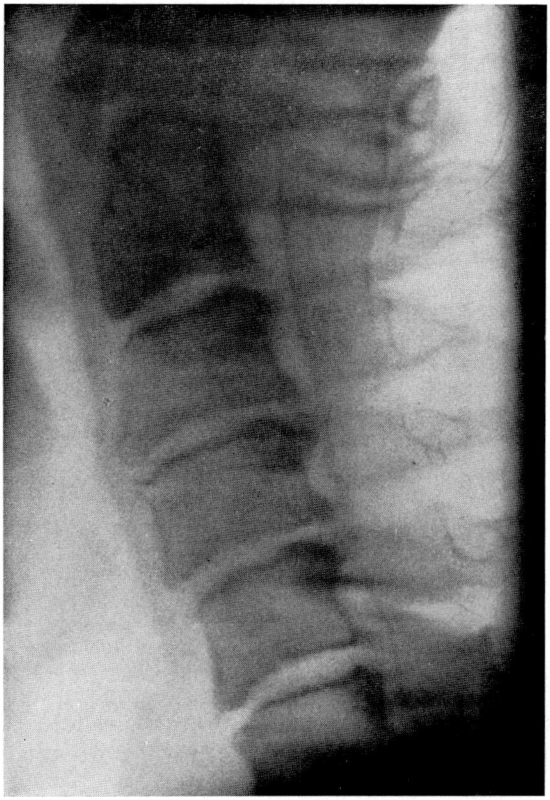

Fig. 11. 45 year old male with slowly progressive Brown-Séquard syndrome. Disc degeneration at the C_3–C_4, C_4–C_5 and C_5–C_6 level. CSF normal. Myelography with tomography reveals that pinching is likely at C_3–C_4 and C_4–C_5 and possibly also at C_5–C_6. Case for laminectomy, not for anterior fusion

nates all dynamic factors. Laminectomy does not prevent stretching of the cord during flexion and anterior procedures are insufficient in cases with diffuse stenosis.

Laminectomy should be considered in cases with multiple level degeneration and a functional narrow sagittal diameter of the canal at more than 2 levels (Fig. 11).

Laminectomy eliminates dorsal compressive factors active during extension of the cervical spine. With laminectomy however, it is impossible to reduce kyphotic angulation, to resect large disc protrusions and to prevent harmful flexion movements and abnormal postoperative flexion movements.

The results of laminectomy of 2 to 5 arches and section of the dentate ligaments—the common procedure in the 1960's—were often not satisfactory (Epstein *et al.* 1963, 1969, Guidetti and Fortuna 1969, Stoops and King 1965). In many cases this was because the laminectomy was too restricted, not removing all compressive factors (Penning 1968, Rogers 1961). Also too much emphasis was often laid on sectioning of the dentate ligaments, which resulted in inadvertent damage of the cord. The opening of the dura enhances cord-dura adhesions (Adams and Logue 1971). Aboulker *et al.* (1965) and Scoville (1961) introduced the more extensive laminectomy

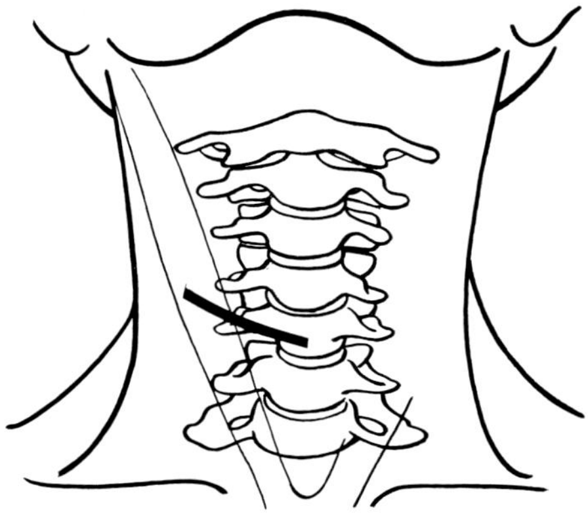

Fig. 12. Skin incision for an anterior fusion C_4–C_5. Others use a left-sided incision. In case of fusion of more than one level, a more oblique incision medial to the sternocleidomastoid muscle is preferable

with (Stoops and King 1965) or without posterior foraminotomy (Fager 1973). According to Adams and Logue (1971) more emphasis should be placed on the reduction of the range of movement of head and neck postoperatively. They advocate the wearing of a collar or brace for some weeks or months postoperatively. Aboulker (1965) had the same goal in mind and completed the procedure by additional sutures of the posterior neck-muscles to get a tough inelastic scar. Gonzalez-Feria (1975) on the other hand demonstrated the possibility of deleterious effects of this scar and tried to counter this by immobilization of the neck postoperatively through the introduction of an additional "crabs plate". Others, like Crandall and Gregorius (1977) are not against opening of the dura and even insert lyophilized dural grafts.

Most surgeons nowadays agree that the anterior approach is indicated in cases with spondylosis at one or two levels, or in cases without demonstrable pincers grip of the cord. The anterior approach (Fig. 12) permits removal of the spurs and allows fusion, either spontaneously or by fusion procedures, like the Cloward technique (Fig. 13 a, b) (Cloward 1958, 1963, Pertuiset *et al.* 1978, Rosomoff and Rossman 1966) or the modified Robinson technique (Fig. 13 c, 14) (Bohlman 1977, Grote *et al.* 1970, Robinson and Smith 1955, Robinson *et al.* 1962, Smith and Robinson 1958, Verbiest 1972). According to Adams (1976) and others simple disc excision gives the same result. He states that the cord is satisfactorily decompressed without removal of osteophytes because spontaneous resorption takes place. Robinson *et al.* (1977) and Bakay (1973) agree in so far that they report that after fusion osteophytes only rarely increase in size, although new osteophytes may develop in adjacent levels above the fused segments. Verbiest (1970, 1977)

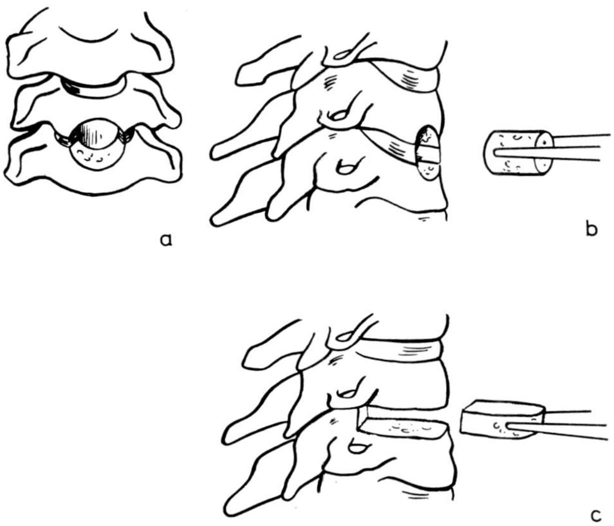

Fig. 13. a) and b) Anterior fusion according to Cloward. A bone dowel obtained from the iliac crest is inserted. For the detailed technical aspects, see Cloward 1958. c) Anterior fusion according to Robinson and Smith. The disc is removed but the endplates of the vertebral bodies are kept intact. Removal of osteophytes through the small disc opening (c) carries the risk of progressive neurological deficit. With the Cloward procedure the osteophytes can be removed with less danger to the cord, but progressive angular kyphosis post-operatively does occur more often than in cases subjected to the Robinson and Smith approach

on the other hand states that in most cases they do not resorb and may even increase in size. The origin of these contradictory views regarding this most important issue is not yet clear. There is no doubt that anterior transdiscal osteophytectomy may lead to progressive cord signs.

Verbiest (1977) *e.g.* reported increase in neurological deficit after medial osteophytectomy in 2 of 39 cases of myelopathy and Crandall and Gregorius (1977) emphasize that anterior approaches in cases with multiple level osteophytes carry the risk of long operations with more laryngeal palsies, tracheostomies and infections, and advice against them. In recent years Verbiest (1972, 1977) and Jung and Kehr (1974) have preferred a lateral approach and removal of the osteophytes through a plane parallel to the anterior border of the canal, not only in cases of radiculopathy or traumatic lateral disc extrusions, but also for myelopathy. According to Verbiest this means a reduced risk of transmission of mechanical energy to the cord. The movement of the chisel with regard to the underlying theca can be controlled by eyesight, which is not possible with the anterior transdisc-space procedure. The uncus is removed and the disc and posterior ridges

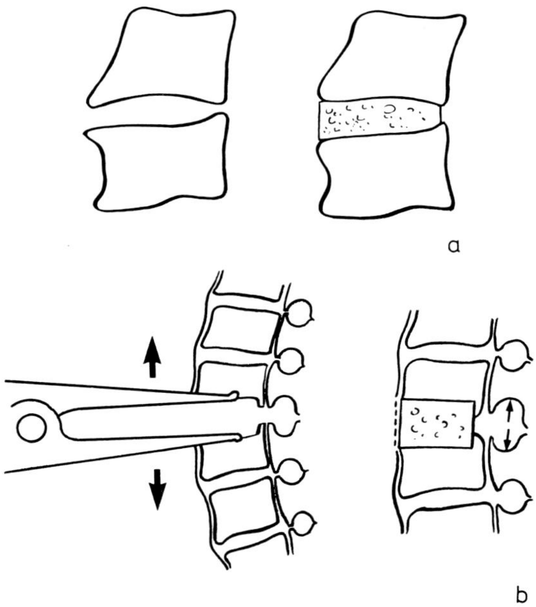

Fig. 14. a) A flattened disc space may—after complete removal of the disc fragments—be brought to normal height by traction in the axis of the spine and the insertion of a tibial or iliac cortical graft with its maximum height anteriorly. b) The same result may be obtained by the insertion of an iliac cortical graft after removal not only of the disc, but also of the adjoining parts of the vertebral bodies. The graft is 3 mm longer than the through in the spine, but can be inserted during manual traction in the axis of the spine or with the use of some kind of spreader. This procedure is more easy to perform than a), but carries the risk of progressive angular kyphosis if the patient is mobilized too early with insufficient external fixation of the spine. It provides good results, however, if the patient is kept in bed postoperatively for 6 weeks before ambulation or is mobilized after 2 weeks and wears a perfectly fitting minerva cast for 8 weeks

excised. The anterior anulus fibrosus is left intact. The operation is completed by the insertion of a small tibial, cortical graft, with its greatest height anteriorly. In this way the original height of the flattened disc space is restored and forward angulation in cases with kyphosis corrected. Graft insertions are not done in case of considerable flattening of the space. Verbiest emphasizes that fusion should be obtained with autogenous tibial cortical grafts instead of iliac grafts after which—also according to Galera and Tovi (1968)—progressive kyphosis may develop. Anterior displacement of the graft cannot occur as the anterior ligaments are kept intact and Verbiest did not observe lateral displacement in 50 cases.

Results of Surgical Therapy

The results of certain surgical approaches which are presented in the literature are influenced by a large number of variables summarized in Table 1 and 2.

On the whole however, authors agree that whatever procedure is performed an operative mortality of 2 to 8% is not uncommon (Clarke and Robinson 1956, Guidetti and Fortuna 1969, Stoops and King 1965). Attempts to compare anterior approaches with laminectomy have been carried out (Dereymaeker *et al.* 1963, Guidetti and Fortuna 1969), but are doomed to fail, unless a randomized therapeutic trial is set up. Results are differently described. Some authors use scales like the one of Nurick or Lees and Turner, others mention percentages of improvement or use terms like good, very good, satisfactory, poor, etc. It is, moreover, difficult to analyse results in relation to the natural progression of the disease.

Table 1. *Variables Influencing Therapeutic Results*

Age of the patient
Preoperative duration of symptoms
Amount and type of neurological deficit
Faulty diagnosis (patient has other cord disease)
Manoeuvres with patient during positioning for operation
Type of operation (see Table 2)
Peroperative cord damage
Postoperative scar formation
Postoperative use of braces
Adequate rehabilitation
Length of follow-up
Observer bias

Generally speaking, however, patients with mild pictures—in which the indication for surgical therapy is least mandatory—usually improve after the operation, whereas the more severe cases—in which the indication is urgent—respond more irregularly (Adams 1976, Crandall and Gregorius 1977, Symon and Lavender 1967).

Return to full function is unusual, except in mild cases. Maximum improvement occurs within the first two years after operation, and laminectomy may reverse the progression of myelopathy, sometimes for a long period. Many worsen, however, when follow-up lengthens. The effect on prognosis of the preoperative duration of symptoms is uncertain. Some authors state that patients with a duration of symptoms less than 12 months have a better prognosis than patients with symptoms more than 12 months. In the latter group the symptoms are often due to irreversible damage to the nerve tracts (Gorter 1974, Guidetti and Fortuna 1969).

The influence of age is also not clear. Some authors observe better results in patients less than 50 years than in those over 50 years (Clarke and

Robinson 1956, Colambert and Pellet 1971, Gorter 1974), others defend the opposite view (Adams 1976). Skilled digital hand function may be partially or completely recover after surgery, but may be worse in as many others. Crandall and Gregorius (1977) did not succeed in predicting success or failure on the basis of preoperative assessment of the most numerous complaints, symptoms or findings.

Worse postoperative results occurred particularly, however, in patients with sphincter loss and lower extremity weakness. The younger the patient, the better his chance of taking his or her position in society and functioning therein (Gorter 1974). If the neck becomes kyphotic during flexion, laminectomy does not remove all causative factors. A low range of postoperative movement may confer benefit. This might explain the marked improvement of some patients shortly after operation, followed by subsequent deterioration (Adams 1976, Adams and Logue 1971).

Table 2. *Variables in Type of Operation Influencing Therapeutic Results*

Laminectomy	extent
	with or without facetectomy
	with or without cutting dentate ligaments
	number of levels
	scar formation
	postoperative angulation
	unwanted retained arch (often C_3)
Anterior approach	with or without resection of spurs
	with or without fusion
	type of fusion
	shape and size of grafts
Lateral approach	type of uncusectomy
	with or without fusion

This means that the end result of operation is somewhat unpredictable, particularly because deterioration may continue as a result of an abnormally large movement range, progressive kyphosis after the operation (Fig. 16) (which occurred in 3 cases of the present author), or an additional osteophytosis at a disc at a higher level. A well-known reason for an unsatisfactory operative result is a retained laminar arch of C_3, which arch is easily overlooked during operation, so that postoperative control pictures should always be taken (Fig. 17). "Natural" deterioration, most probably due to vascular factors may—according to Clarke and Robinson (1956) occur in about 10% of the cases. Some of these patients have amyotrophic lateral sclerosis or other concomitant disease such as an intradural tumor.

Author's Surgical Approach to SM

The author's approach in a case of myelopathy supposed to be SM is as follows: Other disorders of the cord should be excluded, preferably after consultation with an experienced neurologist. The subsequent plain radiographs of the cervical spine include pictures in maximal flexion and extension and sagittal tomograms in extension. The magnification factor can be dealt with by temporarily sticking a marker of 5 cm length to the skin in the midline of the neck (Fig. 9). The natural and functional sagittal diameters are measured at all cervical levels in flexion and in extension. Lumbar puncture is performed with functional manometry (in SM a block in extension is mandatory if laminectomy is to be performed). CSF analysis is obligatory. Myelography with Amipaque, introduced by lateral cervical

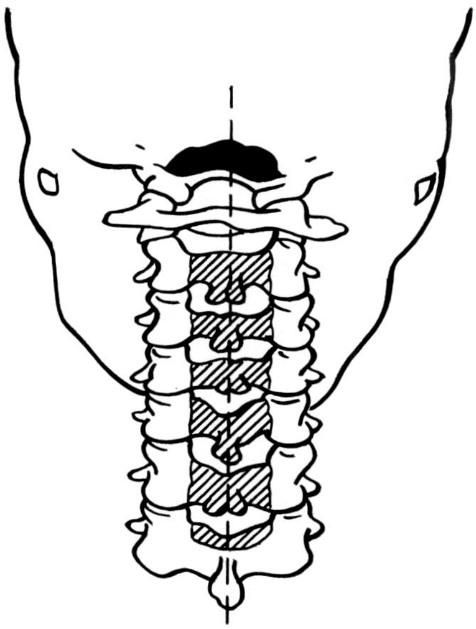

Fig. 15. Laminectomy C_2 to C_6 with inclusion of the upper half of the arch of C_7. The shaded parts of the arches have to be removed. Note that the intervertebral joints and intervertebral capsules are left intact in order to counter the development of postoperative kyphosis

puncture is done in cases of doubt. This doubt is raised if there is no natural stenosis, no local stenosis, no CSF-block in extension, or a high protein content of the CSF.

Laminectomy

In the majority of cases of SM there is a narrowing at three or more levels. Laminectomy usually without foraminotomy and without opening of the dura is then performed.

Technique

Cervical laminectomy in SM does not differ technically from most other laminectomies, although it is usually more extensive. The details of the technique (commonly learned in the early years of neurosurgical training) have been described many times, *e.g.* by Kempe. Some points which in my view are particularly important, will be emphasized here.

The operation may be performed with the patient sitting or prone. In the upright position there is less bleeding, but in our experience, not necessarily better exposure. We prefer the prone position. The extent of the skin incision is determined by the site and number of arches to be removed. It is usually from 3 cm below the posterior occipital protuberance to the spinous process of C_7 (Fig. 15). The incision is continued with the knife until the spinous processes are reached. These processes are identified with the tip of the index finger more than once with an eye on the lateral radiograph. The arch of C_3 is sometimes covered by the caudal end of the spinous process of C_2 and may be easily missed (Fig. 17). The identification should be confirmed by the assistant.

The muscles are freed from the bone close to the spinous process with the use of a knife or a pair of scissors beginning at C_6 or C_7 and then upwards, as the insertion of the muscles on the spinous processes are predominantly in a medial upward direction.

Profuse venous bleeding can usually be avoided if the surgeon follows this policy and strips the muscles from the bone subperiosteally, also from below upwards, and retracts them gently.

Removal of the arches too, is preferably started at C_6 or C_7 and is more easy when the flaval ligaments are opened first and the dura exposed. The inferior lip of the rongeur should not touch the dura. The rongeur should be handled with two hands in such a way that—if it inadvertently slips off the bone—it will not touch the dura or—even worse—press upon the cord. Slipping occurs more often when the arches are removed from above downwards. The cautery is hardly ever necessary. Tamponade of torn epidural veins with absorbable sponges (spongostan, fibrin foam) usually suffices. If coagulation cannot be avoided, a bipolar forceps is used.

Opening of the dura is rarely necessary. In the majority of cases of SM laminectomy C_3–C_6 with inclusion of the lower end of C_2 and the upper half of C_7 is sufficient (Fig. 15). If a preoperative drawing of the anticipated position after laminectomy C_3–C_6 of the posteriorly displaced spinal cord makes a contact with the arch of C_2 unlikely, this arch and the insertions of the muscles on the spinous process of C_2 are better left intact to have less bleeding. At the end of the operation a careful check is necessary to determine whether the arch of C_3 has really been removed.

Fig. 16. Severe arcual cervical kyphosis after laminectomy C_2–C_6 for spondylotic myelopathy. The patient was a rather passive man who—due to misunderstanding—did not get adequate postoperatively physiotherapy and rehabilitation. We proposed a second operation to correct the deformity and to perform anterior fusion C_2–C_6, but the patient refused. He wore a collar for 3 months. Note the progressive formation of bone on the anterior side of the spine, first at the C_5–C_6 and C_6–C_7 level, later also including C_3–C_4 and C_4–C_5. The patient developed a slowly progressive cord syndrome which did not increase any further after 18 months after operation. a) Two months postoperatively. b) Four months postoperatively. The patient wears a collar. c) Ten months postoperatively. d) Eighteen months postoperatively

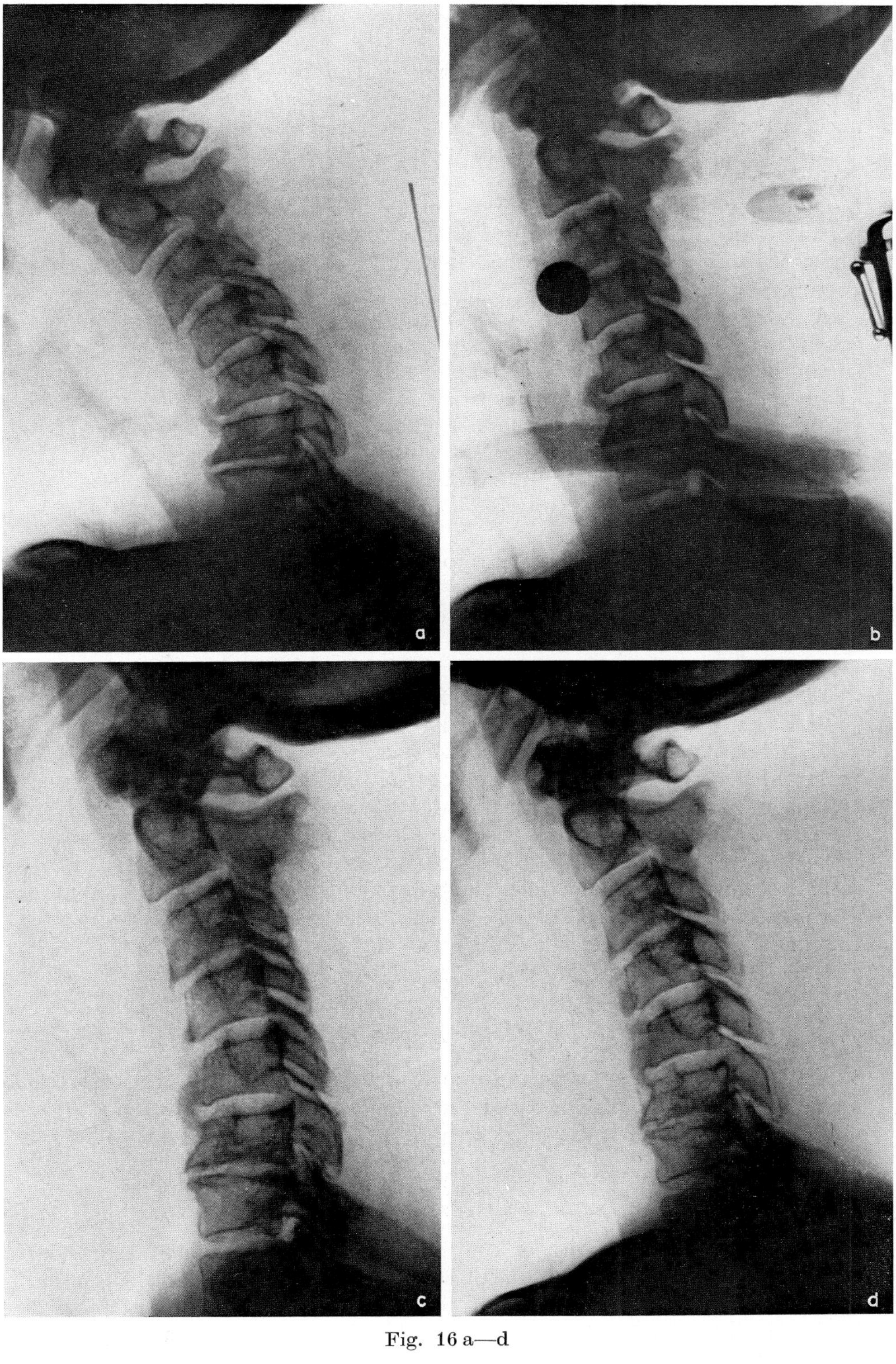

Fig. 16 a—d

Postoperatively the head of the patient can be supported with a flat pillow. Patients during the first days usually prefer to keep their head and neck in flexion, but are taught to keep their head straight up.

The physiotherapist stimulates them to exercise their neck-muscles actively from the second postoperative day onwards. Patients are usually mobilized within 48 hours and go home—if their neurological condition permits—after 10–12 days, provided that longterm out-patient intensive physiotherapy and rehabilitation—which is needed in most cases—has been arranged.

A few days after the operation control-pictures of the cervical spine are taken and some months after the operation flexion/extension studies should be done to give early warning of unwanted instability.

In some patients the preoperative neurological deficit has increased postoperatively either by more root or by more cord involvement. It is usually difficult to identify the exact cause, but common reasons are:

1. Too much flexion or extension of the spine during intubation or positioning of the patient, particularly if the operation is performed in sitting position.
2. Careless turning of patients into their beds after operation.
3. Slipping of the rongeur, which occurs particularly when the operation is well underway and the first two arches have been removed.
4. Use of the rongeur, which is a cutting instrument, as a twisting or breaking forceps.
5. Too far lateral extent of removal of the arches.
6. Use of coagulation, in particular with a unipolar forceps.
7. Attempts to remove paramedian spurs. If, for SM a laminectomy is preferred the spurs should not be attacked.
8. Unnecessary opening of the dura. In most cases the presence of an intradural mass, like a tumor can be adequately excluded by meticulous preoperative myelography.
9. Retaining of the laminar arch C_3 or even C_4 (Fig. 17).

In case of gradual progressive neurological deficit despite operation the diagnosis should be reconsidered. Two of our cases had a meningioma at the atlantal level and two others amyotrophic lateral sclerosis.

Anterior Approach

With demonstrable narrowing due to osteophytes at one or two levels an anterior transdiscal removal of the spurs and/or anterior fusion are the methods of choice. We have no experience with an anterolateral or lateral approach.

Technique

The Robinson and Smith or the Cloward procedure can be performed. We use the Robinson procedure. In both procedures the patient lies supine on the operating table with the neck slightly extended and firmly supported by a padded rest in the nape of the neck. Skull traction, advocated by some authors, is not used. An, optional, right or left transverse skinincision is marked with an eye on the AP plain radiograph or myelogram for the exact level of the diseased disc(s) in relation to the skin (Fig. 12). It reaches from the midline to 2 cm beyond the anterolateral border of the sterno-cleidomastoid muscle. In the case of exposure of two levels a more oblique incision is used medial to the sternocleidomastoid muscle. The platysma is cut in the direction of its fibres. Blunt dissection is done directly beneath this muscle. The line of dissection is just medial to the sternocleidomastoid

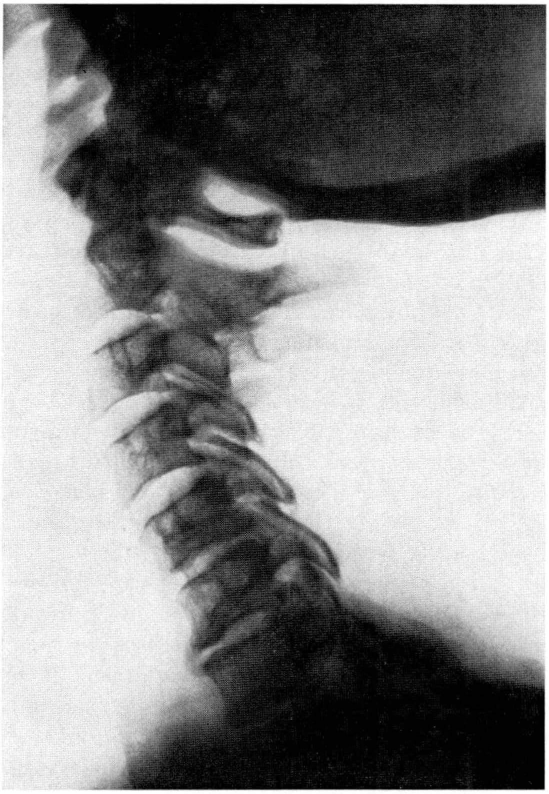

Fig. 17. Cervical laminectomy meant to include the arches C_3, C_4, C_5 and C_6 The postoperative radiograph shows that the arch C_3 was not removed! This occurs more often than is generally thought

with the carotid jugular sheath on the lateral and trachea, pharynx, larynx and esophagus on the medial side. The prevertebral fascia is opened vertically and the vertebral bodies and intervertebral discs are identified. The exact site of the disc is confirmed by placing a radio-opaque marker like a needle in the disc and taking a lateral radiograph or a view through a portable fluoroscopic amplifier.

Discograms are not made. The anterior longitudinal ligament is divided in the midline and scraped off the vertebral bodies with a periosteal elevator.

Anterior osteophytes are removed only if they are extremely prominent. The disc is emptied with the use of a knife, curette, small rongeur or air-drill. Magnification is mandatory. As many authors have reported increased neurological deficit when they tried to remove the posterior osteophytes, we leave them intact and place an iliac or tibial graft in the empty disc space which is spread beforehand. For this purpose a spreader may be used or manual traction on the cervical spine. The graft is tapped home in the disc space, the spreader removed, the anterior longitudinal ligament sutured. The wound is closed in layers with a separate closure of the platysma muscle.

By limiting operative damage to the vertebral bodies and by the use of autogenous tibial cortical grafts, postoperative anterior angulation can be prevented and kyphotic angulations corrected when the smallest vertical diameter is directed towards the spinal canal. These grafts may also be used to restore the original height of a flattened disc space (Fig. 14) and are taken from the antero-lateral surface of the tibia below the tubercle or from the iliac crest with the use of an oscillating saw or hammer and chisel. Most patients with one level fusions can be mobilized after 10 days and wear a well fitting brace for some 4 to 6 weeks. Patients with two level fusions or corrected kyphotic angulations are commonly mobilized after 4 weeks and wear a brace for another few weeks.

Other surgeons consider an intradiscal fusion as too cumbersome and time consuming. They prefer to use a larger graft and perform an anterior inlay fusion covering 2 or 3 vertebral bodies. They do not bother about the destruction of endplates of vertebral bodies (Fig. 14 b).

It has not been proven that this approach is superior or inferior to the intradiscal fusion. In our view the surgeon should stick to the approach which has the best results in his hands. Essential for both procedures is an adequate, not too short period of postoperative immobilization of the spine, either supine in bed or by means of a well fitting external cast.

Some surgeons reject these fusion procedures as posterior osteophytectomy is not done. They do not rely on spontaneous absorption of the spurs which—according to them—does not always occur or proceeds too slowly. For them Cloward's approach is attractive as it gives a more extensive exposure of the osteophytes and herniated discs, which consequently may be removed more easily without damage to the cord. There is no doubt that experienced surgeons may obtain good results with this approach. We have no experience with Cloward's approach or with the lateral approach.

Therapy in Case of Traumatic SM

In the acute stage of a patient with spondylosis, a traumatic cord lesion and no radiological signs of misalignment of the spinal canal conservative management is indicated with the head and neck in midposition. In elderly patients with thoracic kyphosis this usually means support of the head by a small pillow. This positioning should start *in the emergency department*. Skull traction is not indicated.

There is no place for laminectomy in the acute stage, even in case of CSF block, as it has resulted in increasing deficit in the hands of many experienced surgeons (Braakman and Penning 1971, Schneider 1969). The degree and speed of recovery to be anticipated depends on the clinical syndrome. Commonly this is a central cord lesion and then almost all patients are able to walk again after some weeks or months. They may have, however, severe persistent upper extremity involvement.

If—after some weeks—anticipated recovery does not occur the presence or absence of sagittal compression of the cord should be established through postural manometry and myelography. If even in midposition of the neck persistent sagittal cord compression seems likely, decompressive laminectomy may be considered at a later stage and should always be performed in the rare case of progressive myelopathy of which the author has seen only 3 examples.

There are surgeons who prefer a "preventive" surgical decompression or spinal fusion at the appropriate level in patients with transient neurological impairment following slight hyperextension injuries especially in those with a narrow spinal canal and a pincers mechanism (Fig. 8). They fear that any repeat hyperextension injury may cause a recurrence of the neurological symptoms, may be in a more severe form. Particularly in the case of trauma in a narrow spinal canal this is a delicate procedure that carries the risk of a progressive cord lesion so that possible advantages and disadvantages should be carefully weighed. A wide laminectomy may also result in progressive kyphosis, neck complaints and even further damage to the cord. For these reasons we have never carried out such a preventive operation and long term follow-up in over 100 patients meeting these criteria has not proved this approach to be wrong.

Informing the Patient

A most important aspect is extensive preoperative discussion with the patient and his family concerning the nature and the goal of the operation. Many patients expect—when they are not adequately informed—that they will regain their normal power and sensibility within a few days or weeks after the operation and are permanently disappointed when it becomes clear that this does not happen. It should be pointed out to them—*before the operation*—that the goal of the operation is the attempt to stop further deterioration and that improvement may occur, but may also not happen. Short term intensive postoperative physiotherapy and rehabilitation is mandatory as is long term postoperative outpatient follow-up in the more severe cases with permanent handicap to ensure vocational and social readjustment of patient and family.

Acknowledgement

Some figures and radiographs were provided by my good friend L. Penning whose stimulus and cooperation is gratefully acknowledged.

References

Aboulker, J., David, M., Engel, P., Ballivet, J., 1965: Les myélopathies cervicales d'origine rachidienne. Neurochirurgie *11*, 87—198.

Adams, C., 1976: Cervical spondylotic radiculopathy and myelopathy. Handbook of Clinical Neurology, Vol. 26, 97—112.

Adams, C. B. T., Logue, V., 1971: Studies in cervical spondylotic myelopathy. I. Movement of the cervical root, dura and cord, and their relation to the course of the extrathecal roots. Brain *94*, 557—568.

— — 1971: Studies in cervical spondylotic myelopathy. II. The movement and contour of the spine in relation to the neural complications of cervical spondylosis. Brain *94*, 569—586.

— — 1971: Studies in cervical spondylotic myelopathy. III. Some functional effects of operations for cervical spondylotic myelopathy. Brain *94*, 587—594.

Alexander, E., Davis, C. H., Field, Ch., 1958: Hyperextension injuries of the cervical spine. Arch. Neurol. Psych. *79*, 146—150.

Arnold, J. G., 1955: Clinical manifestations of spondylochondrosis (spondylosis) of the cervical spine. Ann. Surg. *141*, 872—889.

Bakay, L., 1973: Postoperative myelography in spondylotic cervical myelopathy. Acta neurochir. (Wien) *28*, 123—133.

Bishara, S. N., 1971: The posterior operations in treatment of cervical spondylosis with myelopathy: a long-term follow-up study. J. Neurol. Neurosurg. Psych. *34*, 393—398.

Bohlman, H. H., 1977: Cervical spondylosis with moderate to severe myelopathy. A report of seventeen cases treated by Robinson anterior cervical discectomy and fusion. Spine *2*, 151—162.

Boysen, E., 1954: The cervical spinal canal in intraspinal expansive processes. Acta radiol. *42*, 101—115.

Braakman, R., Penning, L., 1971: Injuries of the cervical spine. Amsterdam: Excerpta Medica Foundation.

Bradshaw, P., 1957: Some aspects of cervical spondylosis. Quart. J. Med. *26*, 177—208.

Brain, W. R., Northfield, D., Wilkinson, M., 1952: Neurological manifestations of cervical spondylosis. Brain *75*, 187—225.

— Wilkinson, M., 1957: The association of cervical spondylosis and disseminated sclerosis. Brain *80*, 456—478.

— — 1967: Cervical spondylosis and other disorders of the cervical spine. Philadelphia, Pennsylvania: W. B. Saunders Co.

Breig, A., 1960: Biomechanics of the central nervous system. Stockholm: Almqvist & Wiksell.

— El-Nadi, A. F., 1966: Biomechanics of the cervical cord. Relief of contact pressure on and overstretching of the spinal cord. Acta radiol. *4*, 602—624.

— Turnbull, I., Hassler, O., 1966: Effects of mechanical stresses on the spinal cord in cervical spondylosis. A study on fresh cadaver material. J. Neurosurg. *25*, 45—56.

Brooker, A. E. W., Barter, R. W., 1965: Cervical spondylosis: a clinical study with comparative radiology. Brain *88*, 925—936.

Burrows, E. H., 1963: The sagittal diameter of the spinal canal in cervical spondylosis. Clin. Radiol. *14*, 77—86.

Clarke, E., Robinson, P. K., 1956: Cervical myelopathy, a complication of cervical spondylosis. Brain *79*, 483—507.

Cloward, R. B., 1958: The anterior approach for removal of ruptured cervical discs. J. Neurosurg. *15*, 602—617.

— 1963: Lesions of the intervertebral discs and their treatment by interbody fusion methods. The painful disk. Clin. Orthop. *27*, 51—77.

Colambert, P., Pellet, W., 1971: Indications thérapeutiques et résultats opératoires obtenus dans une série de quatre vingts myélopathies par cervicarthrose. Sem. Hop. Paris *47*, 950—952.

Concha, S., Mcqueen, J. D., 1977: Anterior cervical fusions for spondylotic myelopathy. A preliminary report. Spine *2*, 147—150.

Crandall, P. H., Hanafee, W. N., 1964: Cervical spondylotic myelopathy studied by air myelography. Amer. J. Roentgen. *92*, 1260—1269.

— Gregorius, F. K., 1977: Long-term follow-up of surgical treatment of cervical spondylotic myelopathy. Spine *2*, 139—146.

— Batzdorf, U., 1966: Cervical spondylotic myelopathy. J. Neurosurg. *25*, 57—66.

Dereymaeker, A., Ghosez, J. P., Henkes, R., 1963: Le traitement chirurgicale de la discopathie cervicale ; résultats comparés de l'abord postérieure et de l'abord ventrale dans une cinquantaine de cas personels. Neurochirurgie *9*, 13—20.

Epstein, J. A., Carras, R., Lavine, L. S., Epstein, B. S., 1969: The importance of removing osteophytes as part of the surgical treatment of myeloradiculopathy. J. Neurosurg. *30*, 219—225.

— Epstein, B. S., Lavine, L. S., 1963: Cervical spondylotic myelopathy. The syndrome of the narrow canal treated by laminectomy, foraminotomy and removal of the osteophytes. Arch. neurol. *8*, 307—317.

Fager, C. A., 1973: Results of adequate posterior decompression in the relief of spondylotic cervical myelopathy. J. Neurosurg. *38*, 684—693.

Friedenberg, Z. B., Miller, W. T., 1963: Degenerative disc disease of the cervical spine. J. Bone Jt. Surg. *45A*, 1171—1178.

Galera, R., Tovi, D., 1968: Anterior disc excision with interbody fusion in cervical spondylotic myelopathy or rhizopathy. J. Neurosurg. *28*, 305—310.

Gillilan, L. A., 1970: Veins of the spinal cord. Neurology *20*, 860—867.

Gonzalez-Feria, L., 1975: The effect of surgical immobilization after laminectomy in the treatment of advanced cases of cervical spondylotic myelopathy. Acta neurochir. (Wien) *31*, 185—193.

— Peraita-Peraita, P., 1975: Cervical spondylotic myelopathy: a cooperative study. Clin. Neurol. Neurosurg. *1*, 19—33.

Gooding, M. R., 1974: Pathogenesis of myelopathy in cervical spondylosis. Lancet *II*, 1180—1181.

Gorter, K., 1974: Invloed van laminectomie op het beloop van de cervicale myelopathie. Thesis. van Denderen, Groningen.

Grote, W., Bettag, W., Wüllenweber, R., 1970: Technik und Ergebnisse zervikaler Fusionen. Acta neurochir. (Wien) *22*, 1—27.

Guidetti, B., Fortuna, A., 1969: Longterm results of surgical treatment of myelopathy due to cervical spondylosis. J. Neurosurg. *30*, 714—721.

Heinz, E. R., Goldman, R. L., 1972: The role of gas myelography in neuroradiologic diagnosis. Radiology *102*, 629—634.

Hinck, V. C., Sachdev, N. S., 1966: Development stenosis of the cervical spinal canal. Brain *89*, 28—41.

Hoff, J., Nishimura, M., Pitts, L., Vilnis, V., Tuerk, K., Lagger, R., 1977: The role of ischaemia on the pathogenesis of cervical spondylotic myelopathy. Spine *2*, 100—108.

Holt, E. P., 1964: Fallacy of cervical discography. Report of 50 cases in normal subjects. J. A. M. A. *188*, 799—801.

Hughes, J. T., 1966: Pathology of the spinal cord. London: Lloyd Luke.

Jung, A., Kehr, P., 1974: Anterolateral cervical operations using the direct lesional approach. The Cervical Spine, Primary and posttraumatic disorders; Advances in surgical management, pp. 133—146. Bern: H. Huber.

Kahn, E. A., 1947: The role of the dentate ligaments in spinal cord compression and the syndrome of lateral sclerosis. J. Neurosurg. *4*, 191—199.

Kaplan, L., Kennedy, F., 1950: Effect of head posture on manometrics of cerebrospinal fluid in cervical lesions. Brain *73*, 337.

Kempe, L. G., 1970: Operative neurosurgery, Vol. II. Berlin-Heidelberg-New York: Springer.

Lakke, J. P. W. F., 1969: Queckenstedt's test. Thesis, Groningen.

Lees, F., Turner, J. W., 1963: Prognosis of cervical spondylosis. Brit. Med. J. *2*, 1607—1610.

Mair, W. G. P., Druckmann, R., 1953: The pathology of spinal cord lesions and their relation to clinical features in protrusions of the cervical intervertebral disc. Brain *76*, 70.

Mayfield, F. H., 1955: Neurosurgical aspect of cervical trauma. Clinical Neurosurgery, Vol. II. Baltimore: Williams and Wilkins.

Murone, I., 1974: The importance of the sagittal diameters of the cervical spinal canal in relation to spondylosis. J. Bone Jt. Surg. *56B*, 30—36.

Nugent, G. R., 1959: Clinicopathologic correlations in cervical spondylosis. Neurology *9*, 273—281.

Nurick, S., 1972: The pathogenesis of the spinal cord disorder associated with cervical spondylosis. Brain *95*, 87—100.

— 1972: The natural history and the results of surgical treatment of the spinal cord disorders associated with cervical spondylosis. Brain *95*, 101—108.

Nordqvist, L., 1965: The sagittal diameter of the spinal cord and subarachnoid space in different age groups. Acta radiol. (suppl. 227), 1—96.

Ono, K., Ota, H., Tada, K., Hamada, H., Takao, K., 1977: Ossified posterior longitudinal ligament: a clinicopathologic study. Spine *2*, 126—138.

Palleske, H., 1969: Experimental investigations on the regulations of the spinal cord circulation. Acta neurochir. (Wien) *21*, 319—326.

Pallis, C., Jones, A. M., Spillane, J. D., 1954: Cervical spondylosis: Incidence and implications. Brain *77*, 274—289.

Payne, E. E., Spillane, J. D., 1957: The cervical spine: an anatomical study of 70 pe-cimens with special reference to the problem of cervical spondylosis. Brains *80*, 571—596.

Penning, L., 1962: Some aspects of plain radiography of the cervical spine in chronic myelopathy. Neurology *12*, 513—519.

— 1968: Functional pathology of the cervical spine. Amsterdam: Excerpta Medica Foundation.

— Van der Zwaag, P., 1964: Biomechanical aspects of spondylotic myelopathy. Acta radiol. *5*, 1090—1103.

Pertuiset, B., Fohanno, D., Caen, O. L., 1978: Recurrent instability of the cervical spine with neurological implications—Treatment by anterior spinal fusion. Advances and technical standards in neurosurgery, Vol. *5*, pp. 175—211. Wien-New York: Springer.

Reid, J. D., 1960: Ascending nerve roots and tightness of dura mater. a) Ascending nerve roots. J. Neurol. Neurosurg. Psych. *23*, 148—155. b) Effects of flexion-extension movements of the head and spine upon the spinal cord and nerve roots. J. Neurol. Neurosurg. Psych. *23*, 214—221.

Robinson, R. A., Afeiche, N., Dunn, E. J., Northrup, B. E., 1977: Cervical spondylotic myelopathy: Etiology and treatment concepts. Spine *2*, 89—98.

— Smith, G. W., 1955: Anterolateral disc removal and interbody fusion for cervical disc syndrome. Bull. Johns Hopk. Hosp. *96*, 223—224.

— Walker, A. E., Ferlic, D. C., Wiecking, D. K., 1962: The results of anterior interbody fusion of the cervical spine. J. Bone Jt. Surg. *44A*, 1569—1587.

Rogers, L., 1961: The treatment of cervical myelopathy by mobilisation of the cervical cord into an enlarged spinal canal. J. Neurosurg. *18*, 490—492.

Rosomoff, H. L., Rossman, F., 1966: Treatment of cervical spondylosis by anterior cervical diskectomy and fusion. Archs. neurol. (Chicago) *14*, 392—398.

Scoville, W. B., 1961: Cervical spondylosis treated by bilateral facetectomy and laminectomy. J. Neurosurg. *18*, 423—427.

Schneider, R. C., 1969: Trauma to the spine and the spinal cord. In: Correlative neurosurgery. Springfield, Ill.: Ch. C Thomas.

Shimomura, Y., Hukuda, S., 1968: Experimental study of ischemic damage of the cervical spinal cord. J. Neurosurg. *18*, 565—573.

Smith, G. W., Robinson, R. A., 1958: The treatment of certain cervical spine disorders by anterior removal of the intervertebral disc and interbody fusion. J. Bone Jt. Surg. *40A*, 607—624.

Stoltman, H. F., Blackwood, W., 1964: The role of the ligamenta flava in the pathogenesis of myelopathy in cervical spondylosis. Brain *87*, 45—50.

— — 1966: An anatomical study of the role of the dentate ligaments in the cervical spinal canal. J. Neurosurg. *24*, 43—46.

Stoops, W. L., King, R. B., 1965: Chronic myelopathy associated with cervical spondylosis—its response to laminectomy and foraminotomy. J. A. M. A. *192*, 281—284.

Symon, L., Lavender, P., 1967: The surgical treatment of cervical spondylotic myelopathy. Neurology (Minneapolis) *17*, 117—127.

Symonds, C., 1953: Interrelation of trauma and cervical spondylosis in compression of the spinal cord. Lancet *1*, 457—460.

Taylor, A. R., 1953: Mechanism and treatment of spinal cord disorders associated with cervical spondylosis. Lancet *I*, 717—720.

— 1964: Vascular factors in the myelopathy associated with cervical spondylosis. Neurology *14*, 62—68.

Teng, P., 1960: Spondylosis of the cervical spine with compression of the spinal cord and nerve roots. J. Bone Jt. Surg. *42A*, 392—407.

Töndury, G., 1974: Morphology of the cervical spine. The Cervical Spine, Primary and posttraumatic disorders; Advances in surgical management, pp. 14—36. Bern: Hans Huber Publishers.

Tönnis, D., 1961: Über die ischämische Entstehung von Spastik bei traumatischer Rückenmarkschädigungen. Fortschr. Neurol. Psych. *26*, 445.

Verbiest, H., 1970: La chirurgie antérieure et latérale du rachis cervical. Neurochirurgie *16*, 1—212.

— 1972: The management of cervical spondylosis. Clin. Neurosurg. *20*, 262—294.

— 1972: The lateral approach to the cervical spine. Clin. Neurosurg. *20*, 295—306.

— 1977: Personal contributions to the surgery of the anterior and lateral portions of the cervical spine by means of an anterolateral approach. Paper presented at the Dutch "Neurochirurgische Studieclub".

— Paz-y-Geuze, H. D., 1966: Anterolateral surgery for cervical spondylosis in cases of myelopathy or nerve compression. J. Neurosurg. *25*, 611—622.

Wilkinson, M., 1960: The morbid anatomy of cervical spondylosis and myelopathy. Brain *83*, 589—617.

Wilkinson, H. A., Le May, M. L., Ferris, E. J., 1969: Clinical-radiographic correlations in cervical spondylosis. J. Neurosurg. *30*, 213—218.

Wolf, B. S., Khilnani, M., Malis, L., 1956: The sagittal diameter of the bony cervical spinal canal and its significance in cervical spondylosis. J. Mt. Sinai Hosp. *23*, 283—292.

Zülch, K. J., 1954: Mangeldurchblutung an der Grenzzone zweier Gefäßgebiete als Ursache bisher ungeklärter Rückenmarksschädigungen. Dtsch. Z. Nervenheilk. *172*, 81—101.

Tumours of the Posterior Part of the Third Ventricle: Neurosurgical Criteria

F. Isamat

Service of Neurosurgery, Ciudad Sanitaria "Principes de España",
Hospitalet de Llobregat, Barcelona (Spain)

With 5 Figures

Contents

Introduction

Included in this title are the tumours localized within the posterior part of the third ventricle as well as those arising from the pineal region. Pineal region tumours often fill part of the third ventricle and since they may be invasive within the ventricle should not be considered as pure extra-axial neoplasms. Furthermore some neoplasms arising from meninges, vascular and connective tissue within the velum interpositum may involve the cistern and the tela choroidea causing compression of the roof of the posterior part of the third ventricle.

In a 1976 review with Sixto Obrador of Madrid of his and our own material 56 tumours of the pineal region were encountered. Since then 12 more personal cases have been added to this group. They represent 0.7% of all intracranial space-occupying lesions operated upon in this cooperative study. This figure corresponds to the 0.5% to 1% reported in most European and American clinics [Cushing (1932), Grant (1956), Zülch (1956), Olivecrona (1967) and Schmideck (1977)]. In Japanese neurosurgery the proportion seems to be larger, ranging from 8% to 10% of the total of intracranial tumours. There is no consistent explanation for this difference

[Katsura *et al.* (1959), Suzuki and Iwabuchi (1965), Araki and Matsumoto (1969)].

Although neoplasms in this location only represent a small percentage of all intracranial tumours, the central location of the third ventricle within the brain and the relationship of the tumour to vital neural structures and the deep venous system, makes the surgical management of these lesions a formidable challenge to the neurosurgeon.

Since personal experience is usually limited in this type of tumour, the aim of this paper is to present our own experience as well as the most recently published and unpublished contributions on this subject by others, and to put forward neurosurgical criteria for diagnosis and treatment.

Pathological Classification

The confusing nomenclature of the different tumours occurring in this region has been conceptually clarified by Russell and Rubinstein (1959). The three main groups of neoplasms in this location are based on cytogenetic principles. These include tumours of *germ cell origin*, tumours arising from *pineal parenchymal cells* and tumours of *glial cells*. A fourth group of expansive lesions, that may give clinical and surgical problems similar to those described above, are those *extraventricular in the cistern of the velum interpositum*.

Germ cell tumours are the most common posterior third ventricle neoplasms. They account for over 70% of all the reported cases. Two types of neoplasms belong to this group: Germinomas and Teratomas.

Germinomas constitute the most common subgroup of tumours of the pineal region and form 50% of all the neoplasms in this region. They are poorly circumscribed and highly malignant, solid neoplasms. The pineal body is usually destroyed by the tumour. Germinomas are invasive, affecting the wall of the third ventricle and the tectum of the midbrain. They spread through the subarachnoid space and may give rise to extracranial metastases. Intraventricular subependymal seeding, often at a distance from the tumour itself, is a constant finding. Young male adults are particularly affected. This tumour is highly radiosensitive.

Teratomas account for around 20% of the pineal region tumours. They are slow-growing well-differentiated neoplasms with a high incidence in male children. They are circumscribed and encapsulated, may be cystic, and occasionally attain a large volume. Teratomas are benign, can be calcified, do not spread into the subarachnoid space, and are not radiosensitive. They are the only true benign neoplasms in this location, although some histologically malignant forms of teratocarcinomas have been found.

Pineal parenchymal tumours or true Pinealomas are extremely rare. Pineocytomas and Pineoblastomas are the two subdivisions of this group.

Pineocytomas are well differentiated neoplasms that resemble normal pineal gland tissue. They are fairly circumscribed, and usually remain within the posterior part of the third ventricle although some focal invasion can be found in the surrounding structures, such as the thalamus and the colliculi. They seem to be more frequently encountered in young adults than in children. Their radiosensitivity is moderate.

Pineoblastomas are highly invasive and malignant undifferentiated pineal tumours, with a microscopic appearance similar to that of the medulloblastomas. These gelatinous tumours extend into the subarachnoid space and also infiltrate neighbourhood structures such as thalamus, quadrigeminal plate and superior vermis. As with the medulloblastomas, from which histological differentiation can be difficult, they are highly radiosensitive.

1. Germ cell tumours
   A. Germinoma
   B. Teratoma

2. Pineal parenchymal cell tumours
   A. Pineacytoma
   B. Pineoblastoma

3. Glial cell tumours

4. Velum interpositum neoplastic and non-neoplastic conditions
   A. Meningiomas
   B. Cysts
   C. Haemangiopericytomas
   D. Vascular

Fig. 1. Classification of tumours of the posterior third ventricle

Tumours of glial origin: gliomas of the pineal region account for 20% of the neoplasms of this location. Astrocytomas of varying grade are the most common, although other types of gliomas can be found. As a rule they are malignant and thus invasive. Occasionally low grade astrocytomas have been found strictly confined to the pineal. Their radiosensitivity is similar to that of the glioma group elsewhere within the brain.

"Tumours" of the velum interpositum: reports of uncommon space-occupying lesions in this location are occasionally found in the literature. They are lesions arising from blood vessels, connective tissue or meninges. Cavernous haemangiomas, arachnoid and degenerative cysts, meningiomas, haemangiopericytomas and haematomas have been reported. Epidermoid cysts of this region should be included with the cystic teratomas already described.

Diagnosis

Clinical Symptomatology

Tumours arising in the pineal region and posterior third ventricle will compromise, at some stage in their development, adjacent structures. The most frequent symptoms are those of intracranial hypertension due to obstruction of the aqueduct, without special features. Occasionally valvular type headaches are seen as early symptoms. Compression of the superior colliculi and midbrain tectum will give oculomotor disturbances, not necessarily a Parinaud's syndrome, but more often a lack of pupillary accommodation. This the most classical feature of mesencephalic involvement is encountered in less than half of the cases. Midline cerebellar ataxia, dysmetria and hypotonia are seen in patients with upper cerebellar involvement, particularly in cases of pineoblastomas due to their tendency to invade the superior vermis.

We have not seen a single case of pubertas praecox in tumours of this location. It seems that teratomas of the pineal region, and particularly the so-called ectopic pinealomas of the basal anterior third ventricle, are the neoplasms more apt to produce this syndrome. It has been argued that destruction of the normal tissue might remove the inhibitory effect of the gland, believed to be due to melanotonin which exerts an inhibitory effect on sexual development. Diabetes insipidus has been encountered in 10% of the patients and it has been suggested that its presence will indicate seeding of the tumour into the hypothalamic region (Stein 1977), and thus pointing to a malignant infiltrating neoplasm.

Radiology

Plain skull radiographs may show in half of the cases nonspecific changes caused by prolonged intracranial hypertension, particularly at the level of the sella turcica. In addition significant calcification at the level of the pineal gland with changes in its configuration can be seen in some young patients. Calcification of the pineal gland with a diameter of over 10 mm should be considered pathological. Although 60% of the normal population over 20 years of age show pineal gland calcification, this is rarely seen before 10 years of age.

Computerized axial tomography (CAT) is the simplest and most accurate radiological investigation, even at an early stage. CAT scans will demonstrate a tumour which is greater than 100 mm^2 in area situated within the ventricle, as well as the degree of resultant hydrocephalus. Contrast enhancement will be necessary in most of the cases to delineate the mass as well as for differential diagnosis from vascular pathology such as an aneurysm of the vein of Galen. CAT also shows great promise in differentiating invasive malignant germinomas from benign cystic teratomas, but at present, despite this sophisticated method, absolute diagnostic conformation is still lacking.

After computerized tomography, *positive contrast ventriculography* is the most valuable complementary examination. Water-soluble contrast media (Conray, Dimer X and lately Metrizamide) have been used since 1967, without serious ill-effects. This study is performed by catherization of the third ventricle via the foramen of Monro through a frontal burr-hole. In our clinic ventriculograms are now done by permanent placement of an Ommaya reservoir with the distal end of the tube in the third ventricle.

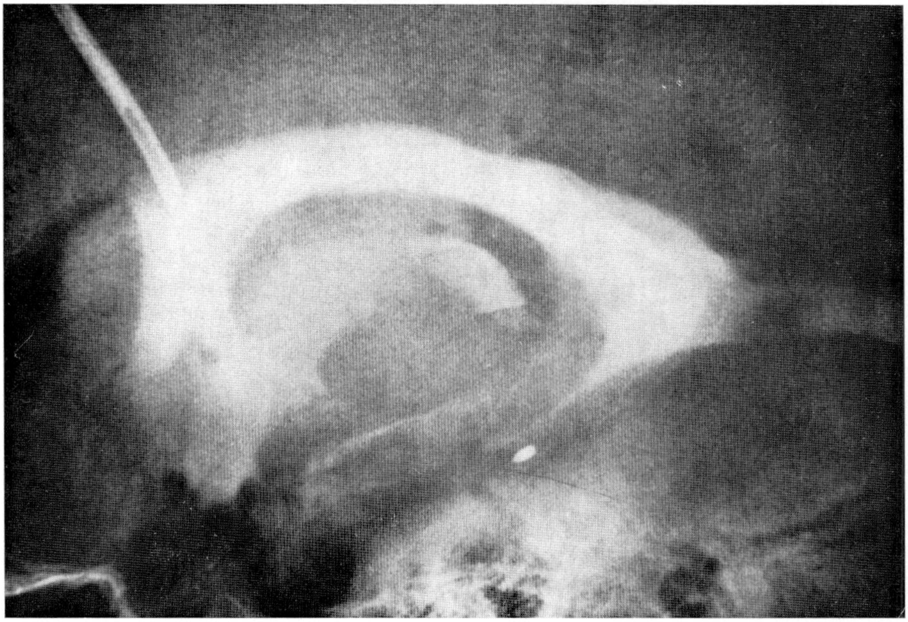

Fig. 2a

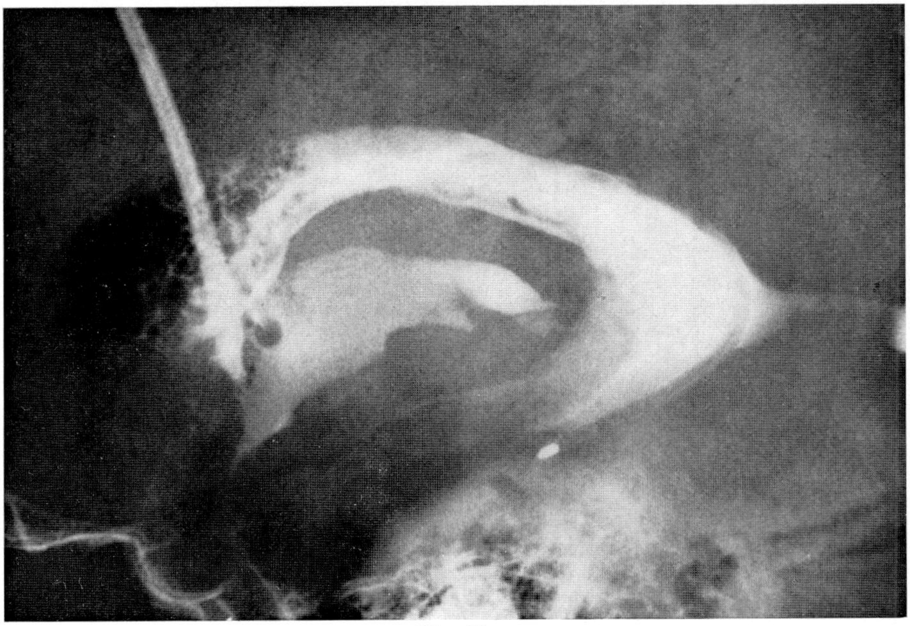

Fig. 2b

Fig. 2 a, b. Favourable result following shunting and radiotherapy (4000 rads). Six years evolution

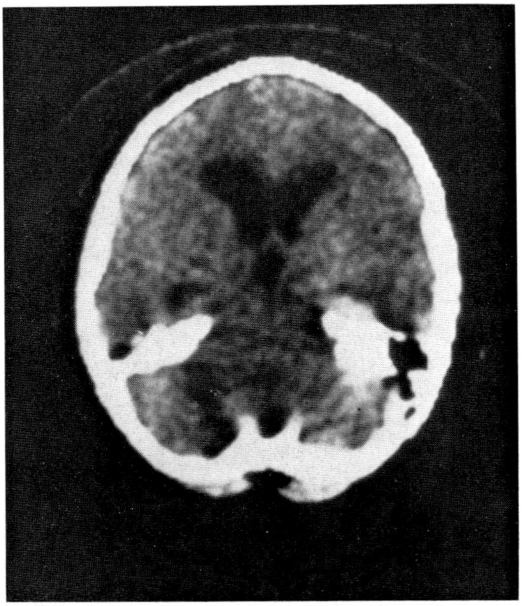

Fig. 3a

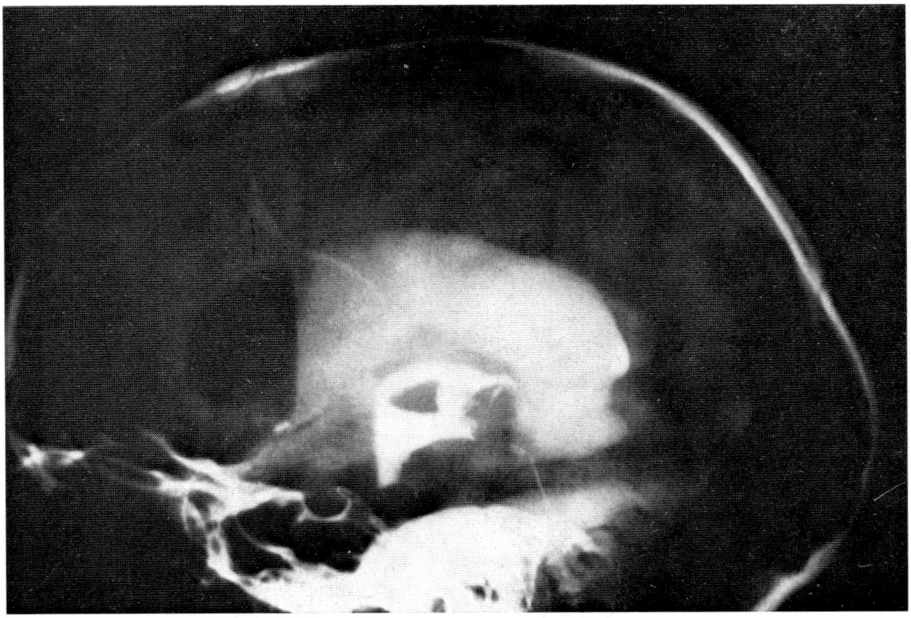

Fig. 3b

Fig. 3 a—d. Malignant evolution of a glioma following ventriculoatrial shunt and radiotherapy. a), b) CAT and Conray ventriculography prior to derivative surgery. c), d) CAT and Conray ventriculography following radiation

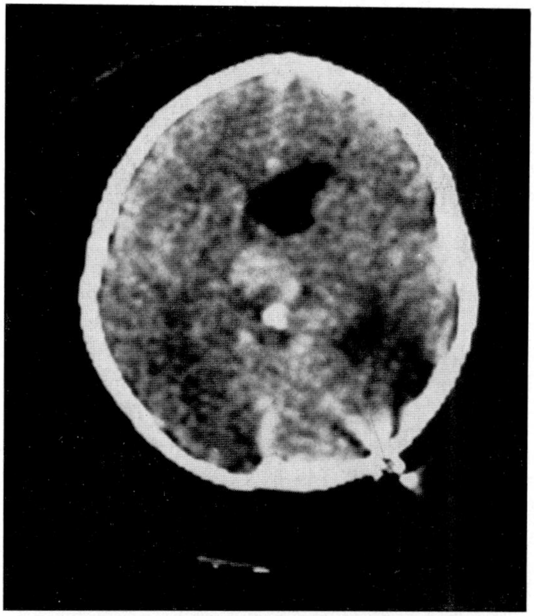

Fig. 3c

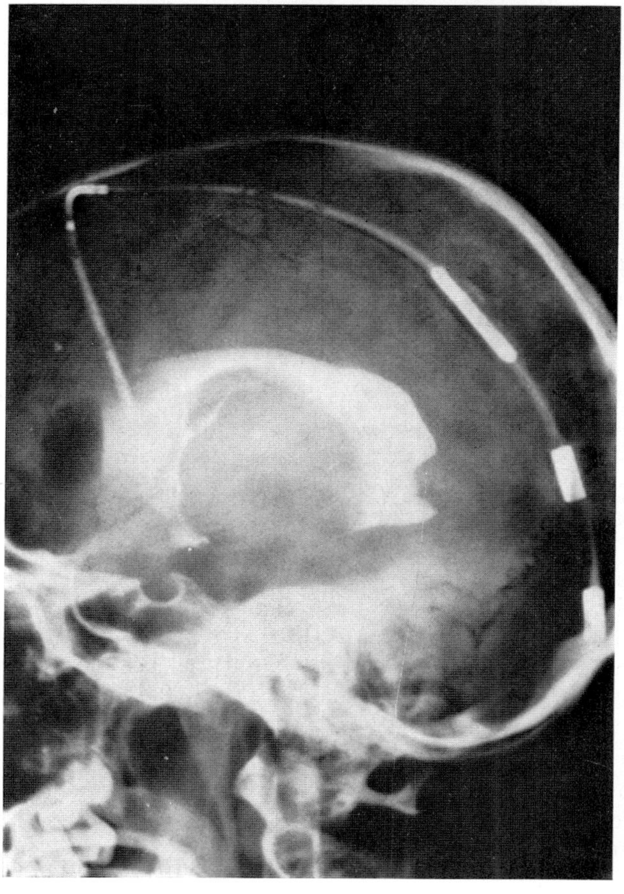

Fig. 3d

Before contrast injection, third ventricle CSF is obtained for cytological investigation. The placement of an Ommaya reservoir also serves for emergency external drainage, if necessary, and for ICP monitoring. With this method, percutaneous ventriculography can be done at any time and shunted patients as well as those subjected to a radical surgical approach, can have routine CAT and ventriculograms as necessary.

The ventriculographic picture is quite characteristic: Amputation of the posterior part of the third ventricle with obstructive hydrocephalus. Anteroposterior tomograms are interesting since non-invasive well-encapsulated benign teratomas seem to give a fairly smooth contour surrounded by a ring of contrast medium, something that is not seen with invasive tumours of the ventricle.

Angiography, although somewhat in decline in the study of tumours of the third ventricle, still has a place in identification of vascular malformation when such pathology is suspected by CAT.

Management

The neurosurgical management of posterior third ventricle tumours has historically been influenced by the earlier unfavourable results following direct surgical approach. Cushing stated in 1932 that he "never succeeded in exposing a pineal tumour sufficiently well to justify an attempt to remove it". The mortality rate was over 70% and the morbidity higher than 60%. This was also the experience of other leading neurosurgeons in spite of different approaches to reach these tumours: transcallosal, Dandy 1921; infratentorial supracerebellar, Krause 1926; transventricular, Van Wagenen 1931, and occipital, Poppen.

CSF Diversionary Procedures and Radiotherapy

Torkildsen (1948) reported a series of 8 patients treated with a ventriculocisternostomy, with only 1 death and no morbidity. Three of them were alive and well 7½, 4½ and 2 years after operation. In the same year Ward and Spurling demonstrated the value of radiotherapy in the treatment of most of these tumours. It is not surprising that a less aggressive attitude was adopted by most neurosurgical clinics. With more sophisticated derivatives of ventriculoatrial procedures and with improved radiation control, shunting and radiotherapy have been considered the proper management for many years. An operative mortality of less than 5% and the many long-term survivals supported this criterion. The five years survival rate is between 60% to 75% of the cases (Obrador *et al.* 1976), with half of them symptom-free. Nonetheless this attitude still leaves untreated the non-radiosensitive neoplasms and benign tumours (20%), and on the other hand carries the risk particularly in children of causing radionecrosis. Although effective in a great number of patients this treatment still remains a "shot in the dark".

Progress in anaesthetics, neurosurgical technique and particularly the introduction of the operating microscope have changed the situation since 1960 particularly in recent years. *Direct surgical attack* has been advocated by some neurosurgeons with some outstanding results (Kunicki 1960, Suzuki and Iwabuchi 1965, Jamieson 1971, Stein 1971, Lapras 1974, Pecker 1966, Obrador and Isamat 1976).

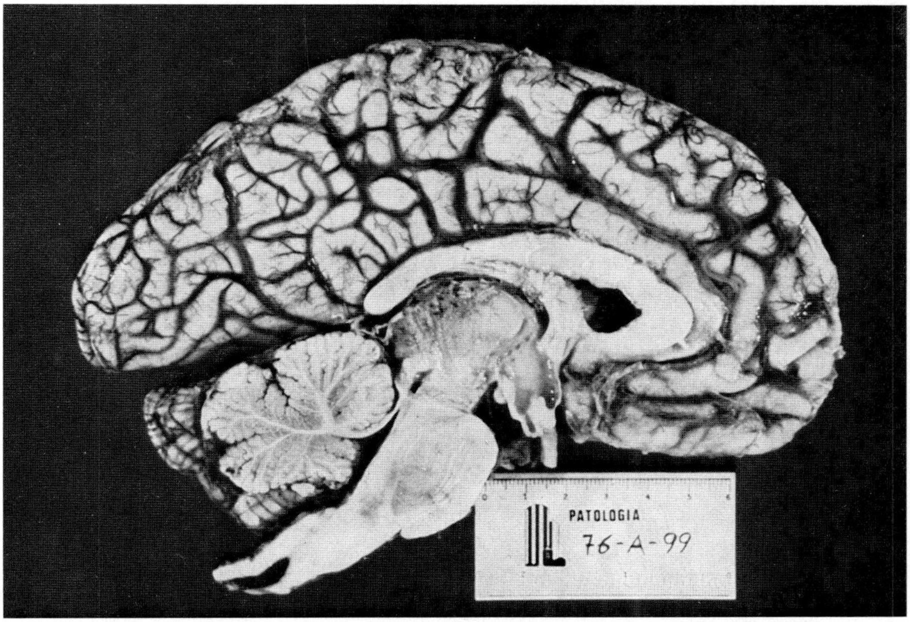

Fig. 4. Pathological specimen of a malignant glioma of the posterior part of the III ventricle

Stein (1971) reintroduced the *supracerebellar infratentorial approach* formerly described by Krause in 1926. The operation is performed in the sitting position with preoperative ventricular drainage. Through a sub-occipital craniectomy extending above the transverse sinus the bridging veins of the upper surface of the cerebellum are severed and the vermis retracted inferiorly. The arachnoid of the quadrigeminal plate is opened using the surgical microscope to expose the tumour and the deep veins surrounding it. Soft or cystic tumours are aspirated and encapsulated ones with loose adhesions can be radically resected. In Stein's experience less than 20% of his patients had a benign lesion, and he reported 1 postoperative death in a series of 17 patients. In a personal series of six cases treated this way there was one postoperative death, a child with a pineoblastoma. Nonetheless the rest of our patients all had malignant infiltrating tumours and were subsequently treated with shunting procedures and radiotherapy.

The supratentorial approaches (Dandy's posterior parietal transcallosal, Van Wagenen's transventricular, and Poppen's occipital-transtentorial) have also had a revival in recent years. In particular the *occipital transtentorial approach* has successfully been used at the present time by Jamieson 1971, Lapras 1974 and Lazar and Clark 1975. This modification of Poppen's technique consists in performing a large osteoplastic occipital craniotomy with the patient in a semisitting position. Following superolateral elevation of the occipital lobe, the tentorium is incised anteriorly from the transverse sinus. The tumour as well as the veins of Galen and of Rosenthal are exposed using the operating microscope. Since 1971 some 30 cases have been operated upon with this technique with a postoperative mortality of around 20%.

A stereotactic approach to tumours of the posterior third ventricle has been used, not only to obtain a biopsy but also to liquefy the neoplasms with a cryoprobe (Conway 1973). Pecker (1974) performed stereotactic biopsy in a series of 14 cases. The biopsy specimens were of good quality in all the cases. There was neither mortality nor morbidity. A similar experience was reported by Sugita (1975).

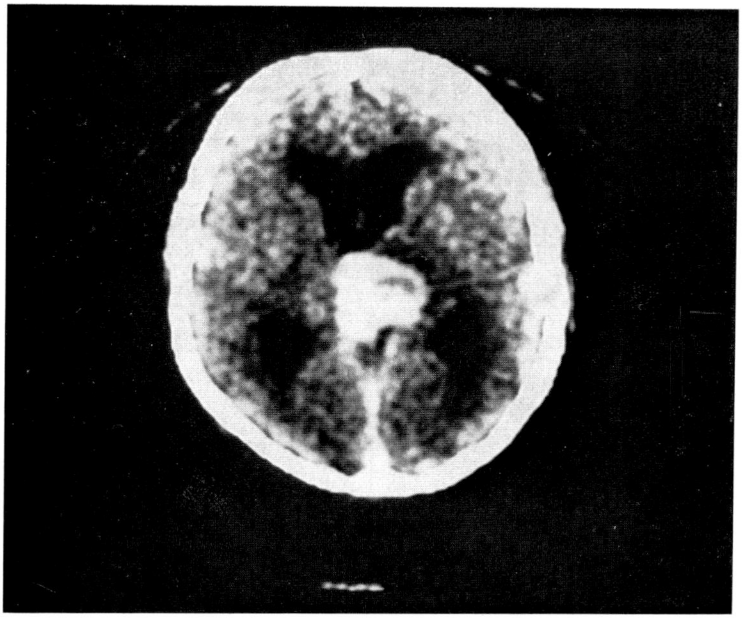

Fig. 5a

Fig. 5 a—c. Teratoma of the third ventricle. a) CAT demonstrating the sharp delineation of the tumour and its cystic component. b) Lateral Conray ventriculography. c) AP Conray ventriculography showing contrast material surrounding the intraventricular bulging of the tumour

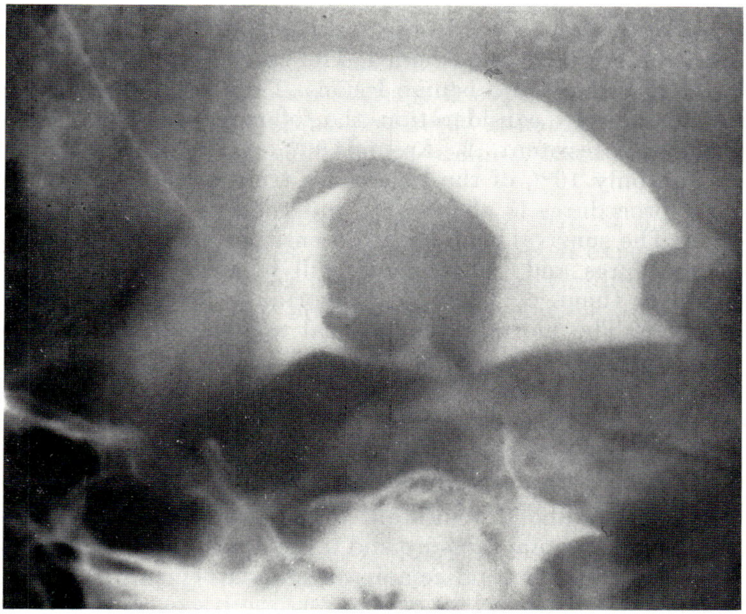

Fig. 5b

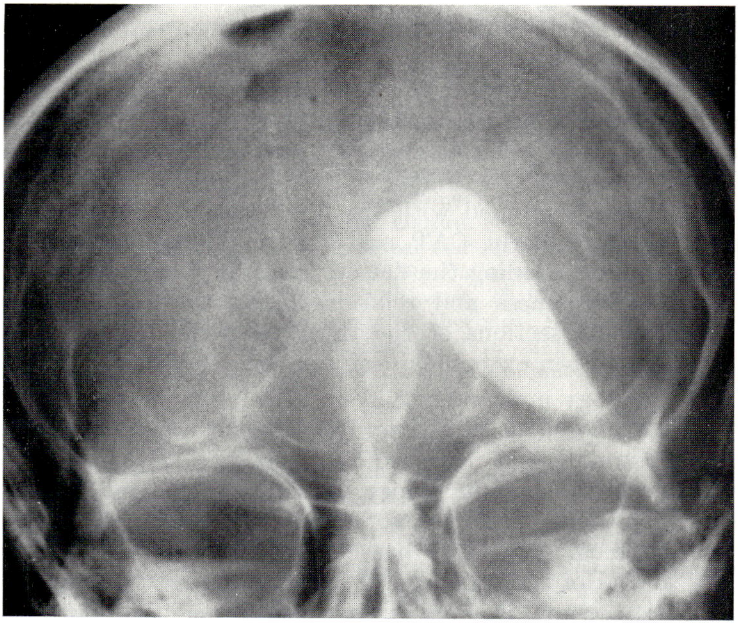

Fig. 5c

19. Pecker, J., Simon, J., Scarabin, J. M., Guy, G., 1974: Application des méthodes stéréotaxiques au diagnostic neuro-radiologique. Neurochirurgie *20*, 5—20.
20. Pecker, J., 1977: Tumours of the pineal region. Jornadas Internacionales de Neurociencias. Barcelona.
21. Poppen, J. L., 1966: The right occipital approach to a pinealoma. J. Neurosurg. *25*, 706—710.
22. Poppen, J. L., Marino, R., Jr., 1968: Pinealomas and tumours of the posterior portion of the third ventricle. J. Neurosurg. *10*, 1—18.
23. Russell, D. S., Rubinstein, L. J., 1972: Pathology of tumours of the nervous system. 3rd ed. London: Arnold.
24. Schmidek, H. H., 1977: Pineal tumours. Paris: Masson.
25. Stein, B. M., 1971: The infratentorial supracerebellar approach to pineal lesions. J. Neurosurg. *35*, 197—202.
26. Stein, B. M., 1977: Supracerebellar approach to pineal region neoplasms. Current Techniques in Operative Neurosurgery. New York: Grune and Stratton.
27. Sugita, K., Matsuga, N., Takaoka, Y., 1975: Stereotaxic exploration of para-third ventricle tumours. Confin. Neurol. *37*, 156—162.
28. Suzuki, J., Iwabuchi, T., 1965: Surgical removal of pineal tumors. J. Neurosurg. *23*, 565—571.
29. Suzuki, J., Hori, S., 1969: Evaluation of radiotherapy of tumors in the pineal region by ventriculographic studies with iodized oil. J. Neurosurg. *30*, 595—603.
30. Suzuki, J., Wada, T., Kowada, M., 1962: Clinical observations in tumors of the pineal region. J. Neurosurg. *19*, 441—445.
31. Van Wagenen, W. P., 1931: A surgical approach for the removal of certain pineal tumours: report of a case. Surg. Gynec. Obstet. *53*, 216—220.

Author Index

Druck: Adolf Holzhausens Nfg., 1070 Wien

Advances and Technical Standards in Neurosurgery

Volume 5

With 78 figures. XII, 224 pages. 1978.

ISBN 3-211-81441-8 (Wien)
ISBN 0-387-81441-8 (New York)

Contents

SPRINGER-VERLAG WIEN NEW YORK